Timer™ DIET

Timer™ DIET

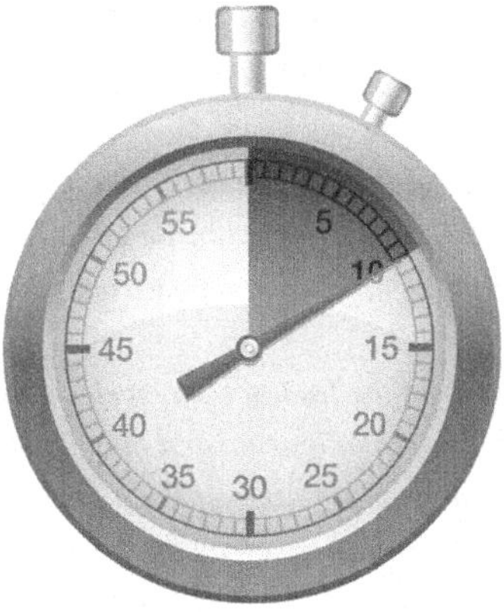

SHERRI SUE FISHER

ARCHWAY PUBLISHING

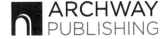

Archway Publishing books may be ordered through booksellers or by contacting:

Archway Publishing
1663 Liberty Drive
Bloomington, IN 47403
www.archwaypublishing.com
1-(888)-242-5904

All of the information is based upon obtaining a physical exam prior to beginning your weight loss program. Be sure to follow your inner guide along with obtaining guidance from your physician.

ISBN: 978-1-4808-0244-5 (sc)
ISBN: 978-1-4808-0246-9 (hc)
ISBN: 978-1-4808-0245-2 (e)

Library of Congress Control Number: 2013917175

Printed in the United States of America

Archway Publishing rev. date: 10/02/2013

To my daughter, Sheilah:

May your star shine forever bright and your smile and laughter never be forgotten.

Acknowledgments

To my two daughters, my two grandsons, and my granddaughter for giving and have given me purpose, which is what we all want and need in life.

Contents

Introduction

How did I decide to write *Timer* DIET? What does the title *Timer* DIET mean? More importantly, how did I come up with the concepts to lose the weight I wanted and keep the weight off?

Before starting this journey, most of my adult life, I was basically insecure with my weight. I cannot count how many times either losing weight or exercising more was on my list of goals for the New Year. There would be times when I gained weight going up a jean size or two, then losing the weight and feeling so excited—only to gain the weight back again. My weight did not appear to pose any *current* health risk and was not a source of concern during any of my physicals—it was a concern for me, however. Prior to deciding to lose the weight for good and maintain my healthy weight, I gained over 30 pounds in a two-year period—I am only 5'2½" tall—I went up five jean sizes in what seemed like the blink of an eye. Once I decided enough was enough and it was time to do *something,* I took out a pad of paper and started writing down what had gone wrong over the last two years.

When I started to write what I thought may have contributed to my weight gain, I truly felt it was all out of my control. It was because I was going through menopause early at 43. I also successfully represented a client in an IRS audit; which lasted three extremely long and stressful years (perhaps that is why I gained so much weight?). Maybe it was because my business was out-of-control and I had *no* time to exercise... there were *so many* other possible reasons. If I needed to eat in order to relieve the stress, and deal with the daily issues at hand, or get some much needed sleep well that was that. Could anyone really blame me for putting on this weight? Besides, I was in my mid-forties; isn't that just what happens? I started to avoid the scale, because I knew there was nothing it was going to say that would help me get through what I was dealing with.

After deciding that the past was not going to dictate my future, I set my goals and decided to press forward...the time had come to decide *how* to lose weight. I had read a lot of books in the past on the subject; it's not like I hadn't lost weight before. I just don't deal well with depravation and diet books telling me what foods I can and cannot eat. Just the thought of someone telling me I cannot eat a certain food makes me crazy (even if it is not something I would normally want). One time I took sugar out of my diet; it seemed simple and healthy enough. The next thing I knew, all I wanted was an espresso with vanilla syrup and biscotti. *Why was I craving this?* Yes, there are times when giving up something is good for you and relatively easy to do. But, what I really needed to figure out was the best way for *me* to lose weight! So I decided to write down what I did not like about all the other times I decided to lose weight or books I read that seemed impossible to follow. Then I reverse-engineered a program that I thought I could live with—keeping in mind the main goal was to keep the weight off for good; so I needed a plan that I could live with *forever.* That is how I ended up with the concepts in *Timer DIET.*

Deciding to write *Timer DIET* came much, much later. A year or so after losing the weight people would ask how I was keeping it off. I started giving my advice via conversations and then e-mails. But, then more advice kept coming into my thoughts as I remembered all that I had done to lose the weight and what I was doing to keep it off—to the point it was bothersome. Ironically, in an effort to stop thinking about the details, I took out a spiral notebook and began writing in it—I had heard if something is bothering you; write it down and you will stop thinking about it; which in a way did happen—the flood gates opened for more memories and thoughts to come to the surface. I had gone through several spiral notebooks over the year since I had started writing. One day I sat down and started reading over all of the notebooks and said to myself, *I think I have a book!* I took an entire weekend and created a twenty-two page outline of all the information that was in the notebooks and color coordinated them into chapters and thus began the book—*Timer DIET.*

I really don't like the word *diet,* but I knew someone would coin it with a diet name if I did not. So you will see—*whether it is when to eat your next meal, how long to workout or to allot for preparing a meal that the timer seems to embody the spirit of the plan, the means to stay focused, and get rid of a lot of the guesswork as to how to do it!* I am so excited to share what I have learned with you; and my wish is that today is the first day of the you, you always knew was possible.

As always…
enjoy the journey!

Sherri Sue Fisher

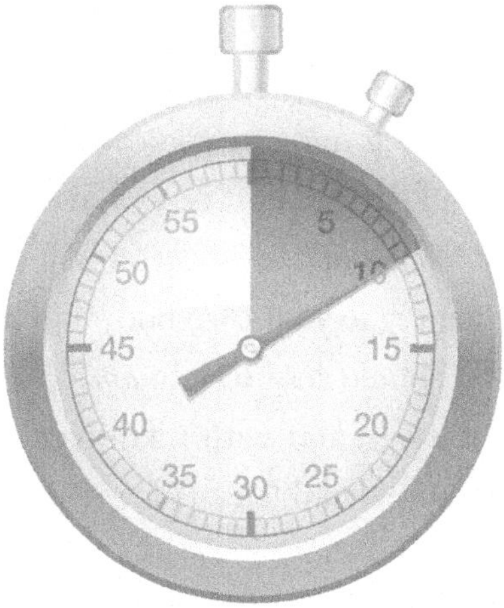

Chapter 1

The Rules and Medical Stuff

The Rules

Have you ever read a book, watched a program, or even bought a piece of exercise equipment with that feeling of *this is it,* only to find out by the end of the book, program, or the instructions there is a catch? Maybe it's a pill or vitamin you have to take or some kind of detoxification that seems frightening. Maybe it's a specific food that is essential to the program you hate, and you feel like saying, "*Why have I wasted my time reading, watching, or buying this?*" I understand. I have been through the same thing and it is frustrating; I want to save you from that frustration—we will go through all of the rules up front, so you know what they are from the very beginning.

First of all, I hate rules, because I feel compelled to follow them, and I feel like a failure when I can't! I think losing weight is probably the hardest thing a person can do—until they actually lose the weight—then keeping it off is. Doesn't sound like a ringing endorsement, does it? Well, don't lose heart. I will do my best to help you understand how listening to your own body and how you feel will be your guide to how you should lose weight *and* keep it off. Having said that, there are a few rules, and with them come some exceptions which I will discuss in more detail later. (I love exceptions!) Here we go:

1. ***You need to eat breakfast within at least 1½ hours upon waking.*** It needs to be a hearty breakfast with dietary fat, protein, and carbohydrates of approximate equal portions—Canadian bacon, an egg over easy, toast with butter, and a small amount of fresh fruit is my favorite! But there are a lot of other options as well, based on foods you already like and know how to make.
2. ***You need to write down every time you eat.*** This is possibly the most difficult rule; yet it will help you the most. You need to keep a record of what you ate and when you ate. *Sometimes* you will want to write down why and how you felt when you ate. Quantities and other details are *not* important.

   The big exceptions are vacations and eating holidays e.g., Thanksgiving, Christmas, and birthdays (yours only—sorry!). I have a lot of ideas to help you with this, including online journaling, texting, apps, and printouts with a binder!

3. ***You will need to eat often throughout the day—approximately every 2–4 hours.*** Whether you set an alarm on your phone, an App, computer widget, or keep an actual timer at your desk; you do not want to let too much time go by without checking

to see how you feel. You will not be required to eat if you are not hungry, and you can always eat before two hours are up if you are. I will give you guidance on how to know if you are truly hungry.

4. ***You will want to include dietary fat, protein, and carbohydrates at each and every meal, snack, or what I call mini-meals.*** Yes, there are some exceptions to this, too.

5. ***You may eat right before you go to bed***—cheddar cheese with saltine crackers or foods with similar attributes.

> *The premise of Timer DIET includes eating primarily cheeses, eggs, meat, poultry, fish, veggies, fruit, bread, saltine crackers, nuts and butter (no sugar-free or fat-free stuff!). Losing weight may be a difficult task if you do not like the majority of these foods.*

6. ***You will need approximately eight hours of sleep at night***—no less than seven hours and no more than nine hours—unless you are catching up. I will go into more detail about this one later.

7. ***You will want to exercise every day!*** It can be any activity with movement that involves exertion. (I hope you notice that I said "want" here instead of "need.")

8. ***You will need to stop eating at the point of satisfaction, not at the point of feeling full.*** My hope is that you never feel full again; it happens to me sometimes still, but very rarely. The hard part of this rule is that you may have to throw food away, because you have reached the point of satisfaction before your plate is empty. Do not eat even one bite more!

9. ***You must enjoy every bite of food you eat.*** If you find you don't like something that you thought you wanted to try, do not

continue to eat it. The program is designed for you to create your own menus based on very broad guidelines.

> *If you have a super-limited amount of foods that you like, it will be harder to get the broad range of foods that will give you variety. Variety makes losing weight less monotonous and helps provide the balance of dietary fat, protein, and carbohydrates needed to lose and maintain your weight.*

10. ***You need to treat yourself from time to time with various things that can or cannot cost money, but don't involve food or drinks!*** Treat yourself to massages, facials, a new outfit, a long bubble bath, a quiet night in front of the fireplace with a glass of champagne—with cheese of course (okay, maybe some food and drinks), read an engaging book, or do whatever your heart desires. These are not meant as rewards for a goal achieved; they are meant to be things to look forward to! Your reward is losing the weight!

Now you have the rules; you can decide whether you want to proceed or not. I think at this point, it is best *not* to make a commitment based just upon reading the rules until you have read everything. I don't want you to feel as if you tried another diet that didn't work! Read through at least *Chapter 5—How to Do It!* and see if it sounds like it will work for you. If there are a few things along the way you want to tweak, but for the most part, you think you are in, then go for it! But, if after reading the rules, you don't think it is your cup of tea, do what you think is best with the book—I truly mean it. My bookshelves are filled with books I wish I hadn't bought, let alone hadn't read. I don't want mine to be in that group. If you are ready to see what *Timer DIET* is all about, let's go forward. I will guide you through each rule, why they are important, and how to accomplish them. I will also show you what you can expect, and what I found helps along the way; so you too, can *enjoy the journey*.

Medical Stuff

This section is very serious. It is not just legalese to cover my butt! You need to get a physical from your doctor. You need to have blood work done and have a thorough examination to rule out any possible health factors before starting any weight loss program.

When you get the results from your doctor, you need to get a copy of those actual lab results for your own records so you can track your progress and see if there are any changes throughout the years you need to be concerned about. You may have to sign paperwork in order to get your results. They may make you come back in person to get them. Whatever obstacle you encounter, just make sure you get your lab results in your hands.

Unfortunately, the labs have a normal range and an abnormal range, and if you are in the normal range—even by 0.01—no warning bells go off, and you are given the all is clear signal. It is important for you to get a copy of your results so you know exactly where you are starting from and if you are close to the abnormal range.

When you meet with your doctor be sure to have your list of questions written down and ready for your visit. One thing to ask about is any medication(s) you are currently on. Your doctor may need to know if you lose weight, since there may be a change required in your dosage of your current medication(s). Ask your doctor at what point in your proposed weight loss you need to be concerned about dosage changes.

See if you are able to talk with your doctor or the assistant before you get your blood work, so you can agree on what to test and why. I found out there are different types of tests according to my insurance company when I went to get my annual physical and asked if I could get my Vitamin D checked. That specific request caused the doctor to say I needed diagnostic blood testing instead of preventive maintenance blood testing and affected the cost of all my blood work—requiring me to pay toward my deductible. Know what your insurance policy allows so you won't be surprised when the bill comes. I found out, if the blood work is taken at my doctor's office and it is preventive maintenance it is completely covered, but if it is taken at an offsite laboratory or is considered diagnostic, then it goes toward my deductible. Knowledge of your particular health insurance coverage is important.

If you don't have health insurance, there are clinics and independent blood work labs that can be reasonably priced based on your economic factors or may be free. See what your options are, and get your physical before you start any weight loss program.

Here are some recommended tests to get. *I cannot provide the normal ranges for you, since they are individual and are prone to change based on your age, weight, and new scientific studies.*

- Alkaline levels
- Vitamin D
- Cholesterol risk
  - Triglycerides
  - HDL
  - LDL
  - Cholesterol
- Thyroid
  - TSH
  - Free T4
  - Free T3
- Liver
- Kidney
- Sodium
- Potassium
- Glucose
- Total protein
- Red blood cells
- White blood cells
- FSH (if you have erratic periods)

In October of 2004, I was diagnosed with—hypothyroidism. I didn't think I had a problem since I did not seem to have any discernible symptoms and I wasn't overweight—a size 4 at the time of my appointment. However, when I went in for my annual physical, my doctor of 15 years noticed a bulge in my neck. We had it tested, and sure enough, I had a thyroid problem, I started taking natural thyroid. I also let my doctor know my periods where pretty erratic, we tested my FSH levels, and it turned out I was also perimenopausal! I was only 42 when I found out; the following year I was in full menopause.

I began to gain my weight a couple of years *after* I started taking thyroid and bio-identical hormones, and I took the same medications while losing the weight using the *Timer DIET* program. I bring this up for full disclosure; lest someone would think I lost weight *because* I started taking thyroid and bio-identical hormones—for me that was not the case. However, having said that, the most important reason to get your annual exam, besides the obvious reason of making sure you are healthy, is to get rid of all the possible reasons for why you have not lost weight in the past. If you know everything there is to know about your body, you can proceed with confidence you are ready to go forward with your weight loss goals.

I don't ask you to do this without knowing that you might not want to know *everything* that is going on inside your body—I get it! I have to say for a person who has gotten a physical almost every year for the last decade, I am always amazed at how apprehensive I am to get my blood work done and see the results. It is almost like opening the envelope for the CPA exam results all over again—I am anxious, excited, and scared. *What if they are bad? What if I didn't pass?* Oh, I know the feeling all too well. All I can say to you is that nothing feels as good as checking that box and saying, "I did it, and I don't have to think about it for another year!" It is a great feeling!

I am not normally inclined to take synthetic drugs. I usually try to find a natural version of what I am prescribed if at all possible. I take melatonin at night if I can't sleep, and since being diagnosed with very low vitamin D—I opted for the natural over the pharmaceutical. I also have taken Ashwagandha for periods of high stress. I use natural thyroid medication rather than synthetic and bio-identical hormones rather than pharmaceuticals. These decisions may need to be made by you as well once you get the results back from your blood work. The best advice I can give you is to research everything. I love *www.webmd.com*. It provides you with information regarding side effects, interactions, natural alternatives, and what to expect with any drug you are prescribed. It also explains blood test results and what each test is meant to determine. Even if you are in the normal range, it is good to know what you had tested and what your results mean.

You may be concerned about not eating as many carbohydrates as many nutritionists recommend. The best test to make sure you are not adversely affecting your protein balance in your body is a quick urine test that will tell you if you have too much protein in your urine. A ketosis test will put your mind at ease and can be done daily if you so choose. If this test is *ever* positive, make an appointment with your doctor as soon as possible, and discuss the situation to see what has occurred. I have never encountered such a situation, but I want to make sure you do not, either.

While I don't recommend high percentages of carbohydrates, as does the Food Pyramid, new USDA Food Plate, or other nutritionists who prescribe percentages as high as 65 percent of your daily caloric intake to be carbohydrates, I think you will find a plentiful amount of fruits and vegetables as well as some bread and saltine crackers *daily* that will insure you are not missing out on adequate carbohydrates. Every meal, snack, or mini-meal ideally should include dietary fat, protein, and carbohydrates.

Overeating, Binging, Purging, and Anorexia

No weight loss book would be complete without addressing the dangers of binge eating and purging, anorexia, bulimia, and excessive exercising (usually preceded or followed by overeating). All of these are serious eating disorders, and they can be triggered by weight loss or the desire to lose weight. If you feel you have any of these issues, even in the slightest sense, reach out to your doctor and ask for guidance. There is no circumstance whatsoever in which purging is safe—not even once.

Accidentally overeating can occur sometimes, just relax, write down what happened and why you think you overate, and then wait a few hours before eating again. However, if you experience any of the more serious issues above—see a professional who can discuss them with you as soon as you are concerned they affect you! Do *not* continue on with this book!

So now you know before you start the program, you will get a physical, find out what your blood work says, and take care of any immediate concerns. Go make that appointment; it can take a while to get in to see the doctor. Let's figure out—*Why Do Diets NOT Work?*

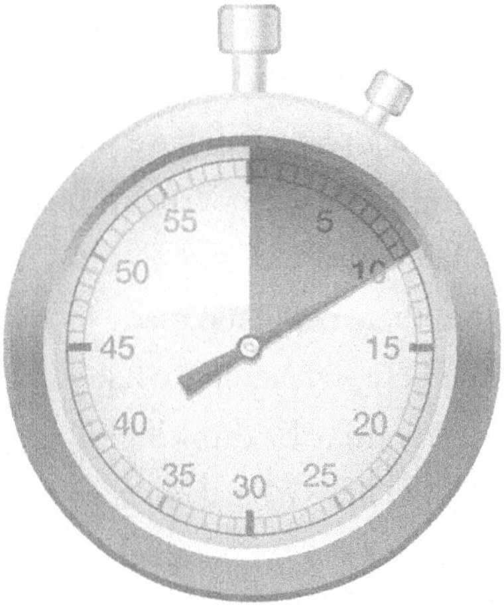

Chapter 2

Why Do Diets NOT Work?

I *think* the main reason most diets do not work is the exact same reason you look to go on a diet! When you are choosing a diet, you want someone to tell you exactly how much to eat, what to eat, and when to eat—so you can be sure you will lose weight and reach your goal. But, here is the problem: *No one* can tell you how much to eat and when to eat, and even though you think it may be easier, you probably feel restricted when someone also tells you exactly what to eat as well.

Part of the fun of being an adult is getting to make choices, and most diets take away those choices. As a result, we do as we are told for a little while. Then we start to resist little by little until we know we are no longer following the regime in the strictest sense and we are no longer dieting. We declare: The diet just did not work for us. It was too hard, too time-consuming, too much of everything a diet stands for. I agree! These issues can be a problem with a lot of programs. Many diet plans require you to eat their foods, or stay within a point system. While other diet plans will have you counting calories, weighing portion sizes, eating specific foods, or eliminating a lot of foods you love. When you look at various diet programs, there appears to be a lot of room to fail, from there being too many foods you might not really like to restrictions on where, when, and what you can eat.

You may be thinking: *If I get to do whatever I want, how is that any different from what I am doing now? How am I going to get any different results if I am free to eat whatever—whenever?* Good question! This is definitely not a do whatever, whenever you want program; it is about learning to listen to your body and what it needs and sometimes what it wants. Your body will actually tell you when it has had enough food and that sensation comes much earlier than when you feel *full*. Also, your body, through trial and error, will tell you what foods it wants to make it feel better; otherwise known as cravings! Not all cravings are bad; it is when you deny those cravings and try to ignore them, you will find that you will eat more of something else in an effort to avoid the simple craving you had in the first place.

When you pick out a food do you think of how it will affect you? Do you incorporate all types of foods into your daily dietary intake? Or, maybe you like a certain food and eat *it* the majority of the time? I am going to show you how to eat until you are just satisfied and not one bite more. We will incorporate different foods in your meal plans while thinking about flavor, texture, and temperature for variety, while maintaining nutritional value. Most importantly, we will discuss how to eat when you have anywhere from a minute to 30 minutes to prepare your meal; when you are at a restaurant, fast food place, on a date, at a family event, or eating at home; and when you are cooking for yourself or an entire group of family and friends.

Your feelings about exercise can be a hindrance when it comes to losing weight. Have you ever looked at how many calories you burned off at the gym only to decide you *earned* the right to eat something—something sweet? I know I have! If you eat something sweet without offsetting it with dietary fat and protein, you are going to increase your blood sugar and thus your cortisol levels, which have been attributed to weight gain. It is fine to eat after workouts just make sure what you eat includes all three: dietary fat, protein, and carbohydrates.

Maybe you were told to workout three times a week. Have you ever gone an entire week only to find you never found *the* three days for you to go workout? If you don't commit to working out on a daily basis it is going to be easy to put it off. When I was young, I spent the summers with my grandparents and my grandpa took us kids for a walk *every* night after dinner. It was fun! Those walks after dinner are some of the best memories I have of our time together.

Exercise is really for so much more than losing weight: it relaxes you, helps you sleep better, and helps tone your muscles. Aerobic exercise is also a great stress reliever. I started getting on the treadmill for 20 minutes whenever I was having a stressful time with one of my clients; that alone increased how often I worked out. As a bonus, I was able to get back on the phone with the client and be calm about the situation. I understand this may not be an option for everyone, but even if you are allowed a 15 minute break, you can use it to reenergize and refuel yourself and be more productive when you return to work—even if it means just taking a walk around the building while grabbing a mini-meal from *your* menu plan.

You will want to create a place where you can workout at home, you can have a gym membership if you want, but everyone needs a home gym. I will show you three different types of home gyms to choose from. One which costs no money at all; you can exercise in your home as it is right now using only your body and various pieces of furniture. Another with minimal costs, less than $250, and is portable, so you can put it in your closet. There is also the option of turning one of your rooms into a workout center. The whole idea is to get rid of any reasons for not working out. We do not want to let weather, time, nor insecurities deter us from working out.

While we are on the topic of exercise, there is also the reverse possibility when it comes to deciding on whether to exercise or not and that is: You may realize you are hardly burning any meaningful calories—so why bother exercising? You may say to yourself, *I just won't eat dessert,* or *I will skip the pasta at dinner,* or *maybe I will forego that bottle of wine.* That philosophy won't work. The health benefits of exercise just cannot be replaced by eating or drinking less. Can you lose weight and not exercise? Sure. Should you? Absolutely not! I don't recommend looking at the calorie counter on the machines at all. When I saw I was only burning 150 calories over a 30 minute period, I was in shock. I could eat 150 calories easily. I just stopped looking at it. Most of the time, my cell phone covers it, or I just tune it out.

Another reason some diets don't work is that they don't acknowledge the importance of dietary fat which helps you feel satisfied. Without dietary fat at each meal or mini-meal there is a tendency to overeat. Dietary fat is also important for your skin, hair, nails, and every part of your body. It is unfortunate that dietary fat has gotten such a bad name when excess weight is really the problem. I prefer the term *dietary fat* so as to remove the negative connotations associated with the word *fat.*

Have you ever tried to overeat steak? It is not very easy. What about a bag of potato chips? That's pretty easy to do. This is because potato chips are mostly carbohydrates. It is much easier to overeat carbohydrates than it is to overeat dietary fat with protein. When I select meals or mini-meals, I look for combinations that include dietary fat, protein, and carbohydrates. The ratio can change from meal to meal, but I always try to get them somewhat close. I don't use a lot of math or measuring; instead, I have learned to read a label pretty quickly. I know the basics: most meat is dietary fat and protein, so I need carbohydrates with it. I also know that most vegetables and fruit are primarily carbohydrates, so I need to pair them up with protein and dietary fat like beef, fish, poultry, or dairy. It is not very complicated once you know how to read a label in just 15 seconds—it just takes a little practice.

Another problem I have seen with other diets is the idea of *calories in and calories out*. I have no idea how this can possibly be 100 percent true. Just try a couple of things for me, and see if you still believe in *calories in and calories out*. Weigh a gallon of water on the scale—*do not drink it; drinking too much of anything can kill you*—it weighs about eight pounds, yet it has zero calories. Next, weigh yourself right before you go to bed (just this once) and then again the next morning; I bet you lost one to three pounds and you did not run a marathon during the night. These are a couple of the theoretical problems I have with *calories in and calories out*. Bottom line: Do not worry about calories in or calories out—they are not a part of the *Timer DIET* program.

However, there is *some* value in looking at calories; they can be anecdotal for comparison and contrast. For example, when I compare two frozen dinners, I would check the ratio of dietary fat, protein, and carbohydrates. If one dinner had 5 g (grams) of dietary fat, 10 g of protein, and 25 g of carbohydrates while another dinner had 10 g of dietary fat, 10 g of protein, and 15 g of carbohydrates, I would pick the second one, because the numbers are closer to each other. I might not focus on how many calories there are since I know I would only eat until I felt satisfied and no more; but I may want to compare the two and see if they are somewhat equal. In the case above the first dinner would have 185 calories, and the second one (the one I selected) would have 190 calories—so they are similar. The *Timer DIET* program is based on the ratio of grams not the ratio of calories of dietary fat, protein, and carbohydrates.

Focusing on fiber is another concept that does not make sense to me. Fiber is a type of carbohydrate—all three components (dietary fat, protein, and carbohydrates) work together, and to eliminate or minimize any one of them for a meal will cause you to feel out of sorts. This brings up a saying that I find misleading: eat your fruits and vegetables. It is an incomplete saying. While fruits and vegetables are important and are a great source of fiber, most of them are primarily carbohydrates (*there are some which do have substantial sources of protein—beans and dietary fat*—olives). So eat your fruits and vegetables and be sure to add some dietary fat and protein to them, if needed!

This may be the biggest reason of all as to why diets don't work in the long run: Because we don't know when it is time to stop and maintain or for that matter, how! There is so much focus on losing weight we lose sight of when we should stop and maintain. Never mind that *everyone* wants to chime in as to when we have and have not lost enough weight; it can drive a person crazy. More than likely, other people's comments will just get you off track and cause you to lose direction if you haven't already decided for yourself when *you* are ready to move over to maintaining.

Sometimes when we diet, our goal is to lose weight for a wedding or special event. So we do. Then what? We gain it back, because there was no plan for maintaining. It can be even more insidious than that. You actually get more affirmation from the public when you are losing or have just lost weight. Once you have kept it off for a few months, people stop talking about it. You begin to miss the positive reinforcement you once had from the outside world. It can be a letdown. I will go over all of this and more, including a cathartic activity in the last chapter of your journey, *(Chapter 9—Now that You Have Lost the Weight)* that will help you in your transition to maintaining and minimize the chance you will put the excess weight back on.

Involving others in your weight loss journey or plan may actually prevent you from achieving your weight loss goal. I know you have heard all about finding a partner to workout with and be accountable to, but I don't think this approach always works. What if your friend loses weight faster than you? What if your friend constantly questions your food choices or how much you eat? It can strain a relationship when you have made yourself accountable to someone you are close to.

I feel losing weight is a solo project—so much so I recommend you do not tell anyone you are in the process of losing weight. Let others tell you that you have lost weight. I am not sure how the topic of including a friend or partner in your weight loss plan even happens. You would not tell someone else they need to lose weight, would you? Please don't. Everyone has their own journey. You may be an inspiration, but don't ask someone else to do something they may not be ready for.

Another thing that may prevent you from keeping the excess weight off for good is that you are doing something to lose weight you most likely will not be doing for the rest of your life. While there is a significant mental transition period between losing weight and maintaining, there really isn't a lot of difference between what I used to do when I was losing weight and what I do now that I am maintaining. There are slight differences, like exercising a *little* less and including a *little* more alcohol or dessert a *little* more often, but nothing major. However, if you are on a strict diet and you commit to it because you want to lose weight, what will you do when you have reached your goal? There will come a time when it is just too much effort to continue on *forever* or worse, maybe you are on a type of diet you are only supposed to do for a few weeks to lose weight really fast, which I do not recommend. If you take nothing else away from this book, remember this:

> ***If what you are doing to lose weight, you are not willing or able to do for the rest of your life, you are not going to be keeping the weight off for very long!!***

This brings us to another problem with many weight loss plans: they require a pill, powder, or something special you need to do. You obviously do not want to do this forever and when you stop, the weight will more than likely come back. This may or may not be only because you have associated your weight loss with the pill, powder, or special thing you did. Most importantly, you will not associate your weight loss with you! Conversely, if you know *you* were the primary reason for losing weight that sense of accomplishment will stay with you forever and help you with the change over from losing weight to maintaining.

Last but not least, food portions are a huge reason diets do not work. How many diets tell you the exact portions they think you should eat? Almost all of them. So I have good news and bad news. The bad news is I will not be able to tell you how much to eat at each meal; the good news is you will begin to listen to your body and it will tell you how much to eat at each and every single meal or mini-meal. If you think about it realistically, if someone is telling you how much to eat, then you are no longer listening to your body and what it needs. You may actually eat more at a meal than you feel comfortable with, because that is what you are told to do.

> *I remember one diet I read said I was supposed to have a half cup of oatmeal, a glass of skim milk, half a grapefruit, a hard-boiled egg, and slice of dry toast for breakfast. I was stuffed! This is not good.*
>
> *If you are full, then your stomach is stretching. If your stomach is stretching, the next time you eat, it will need more food before it feels full. Therefore, it is so important to not go for the feeling of full, instead go for just satisfied.*

The alternative to diets having you eat too much is not providing you with enough to eat at each meal; so you are on pins and needles, waiting for the next time you *get* to eat or feeling like a failure because you gave in and ate *something—anything.* When we give in and decide to eat something, it is usually something we would not eat if we were thinking more clearly.

So promise yourself right now and say this with all your heart:

I will not go on a restrictive diet ever again! I will learn what is best for me and let my inner self be my guide!

We will go over all the ways to help you recognize when you are satisfied yet not full so you can go 2–4 hours without food and be ready for your next meal without feeling ravenous or the need to continually eat throughout the day. We will also go over possible reasons you may feel like you want to eat but are not hungry and aren't sure exactly why or what to do about it. But first, we need to figure out—*Why Do YOU Want to Lose Weight*?

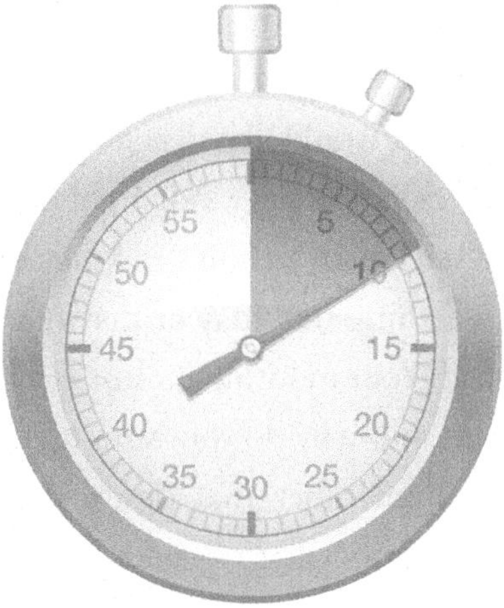

Chapter 3

Why Do *You* Want to Lose Weight?

So why do you want to lose weight? How much weight do you want to lose? Why did you buy a book on losing weight? Have you thought about your goals? Have you ever been at the weight/size you want to be? How long ago was it? Do you want to keep the weight off after you lose it? This last question may sound odd, but what if you really only want to lose weight for an event. Are you thinking about after the event? Are you prepared for all that goes into losing weight? Have you considered the cost of clothes, people's comments, people wishing that you fail and gain the weight back (sad but true), people hoping that you never succeed (even sadder but true). Have you thought about your own feelings about your body after you lose the weight? (There are A-list actresses who think that their bodies are less than perfect? When we all would agree they are amazing!)

There are many reasons to want to lose weight. It is important to decide what your reasons are before you start your weight loss program. While I would like to believe that health is one of them, we all know of a person whose grandparent died from the effects of smoking but just weren't ready to quit smoking themselves. We are just not motivated by something that may or may not happen to us 25 to 40 years down the road. Your motivation must be now!!! What do you want to accomplish *now*, and why do you want it, *now?*

Remember that desire is not motivation, and motivation does not require desire—both together are great, but motivation is more important than desire. Actors have motivation! If they don't get their bodies back in shape after having a baby, they start to lose the roles they are used to getting. Their weight affects their moneymaking ability—now that is motivation. The same goes with weight loss spokespersons; they have huge amounts of motivation—money.

What can you do to motivate yourself (assuming no one will pay you if you do or fire you if you don't)? Look for a feeling. Ask yourself: *How do I feel now? How do I want to feel? What do I need to do to feel that way?* Now think about how your life will be once you lose the weight. How will you feel? What will you look like? What kind of clothes will you be wearing? What type of activities will you be doing? What kind of comments will you hear? Visualize a different you. How does it feel?

Start a journal (nothing fancy required) and write down all the reasons you want to lose weight. They can be flimsy, selfish, crazy, and so unrealistic that someone else would laugh, but it doesn't matter! This is a list for you alone, so just keep listing your reasons—all of them. Go through them one by one and see which ones actually tug at your heart when you read them, make you giddy, or make you smile so big that you can't stop. Circle those. They are the reasons you want to remember when you wonder why you are doing this and if it is worth it to make changes in your life.

Motivation is the most important thing in any goal. Inward motivation is what will sustain you through the rough patches. Outward motivation may give you the spark to get you started. No one needs to know or question what motivates you! Your motivation is yours and yours alone. It can be vanity or a more serious issue such as a health crisis, or wanting to avoid a health scare. Whatever your motivation is: own it, cherish it, and be thankful for it. Above all, do not let anyone else tell you that you need to lose weight because you are not sexy enough. Sexy is a state of mind and anyone can be sexy regardless of how much they weigh.

This may seem like an odd time to bring up the downside of losing weight, but before I have you go too far into, *why you want to lose weight*, let's talk about the reality of it. Not everyone in your life wants you to lose weight. They may not tell you this, but there are different reasons for their lack of enthusiasm for your plan. Some people like things just the way they are. Some of your friends or partner may wonder if you will still want to be with them after you have lost weight. This is tricky since your motivation *may be* to attract a new partner…which is fine, but you may get some resistance—for obvious reasons.

There are other reasons people may not want you to succeed. Others may have tried to lose weight and were not successful; they just determined it was too hard. If you do it, then their rationalization just got a little questionable. Maybe a thin person in your life will not be happy, because they are used to all of the attention and they may have to start sharing it with you. Keep in mind that other people's resistance is just that: their resistance. Don't ask them about it; don't comment about it; do not even worry about it. More than likely, they don't even realize they feel the way that they do. Just recognize that it may occur so you are not caught off guard when they bring your favorite cupcakes into the office or throw a party without one healthy thing to eat. In my case it was my mom who sent me blueberry pancakes with syrup from a gourmet delivery company for the first Christmas after I had lost 25 pounds, and the next year, she sent me a deep-dish chocolate espresso cake. I just called and said, "Thank you so much." You may need to smile and say, "I love it! How did you know?" and give it to someone else. I gave the blueberry pancakes to my client's wife, who was pregnant with twins and needed to gain some weight—per her doctor's orders—and therefore could easily afford the extra calories. I never asked her if she liked them; she may have given them to someone else!

Then there are going to be the people who tell you there is a better, faster, or more efficient way to lose weight or ask you how much more you are going to lose when you thought you were almost there! Yes, then there is the infamous, "Let me give you my personal trainer's card. He can help you firm up." Yikes! Everyone has an opinion on the subject. My client actually said, "We should go golfing again soon—this time we can *walk* the course." To which I laughed hysterically, "I don't think so! It is 110 degrees outside!" Just try to be as graceful as possible and stick to what you feel is right for you; but sometimes people do have helpful ideas; so just listening can't hurt.

So more bad news: you are going to be the same you after you lose weight as you were before you lost weight unless you do some soul-searching during the process—which I highly encourage. It is a great time to figure you out! What makes you—you? If you were someone else looking at yourself, what would you like to be different in the way you are with others and most importantly how you are with yourself. Sometimes we are so hard on ourselves that it really starts to affect our self-worth, creating stress and making it even more difficult to lose weight. My caution is that if one of your motivators is to have a better social life and have people be more attracted to you, losing weight may not be the only thing you will want to work on right now. There are plenty of overweight women with amazingly hot, wealthy husbands, careers to be envied and plentiful friends. My point is: you may feel it is your weight that is setting you back, when in fact it is not.

Losing weight is a solo project. Do not ask your spouse, sisters, or friends if they want to lose weight with you! That is just not a nice thing to do! You wouldn't want someone to ask you to lose weight with them, if you were not ready. If the subject comes up *after* you have been losing weight and people start to notice and ask if they can join you on a hike or a walk, say, "Sure." (Reminder: You aren't going to admit that you are losing weight until you have lost about 10 pounds!)

Only give pointers if others ask for them! Keep it simple, and say something like, "I eat often in smaller amounts." After reading this book, you will find there is a lot that goes into losing weight, and if you are prepared, it can go pretty smoothly. But everyone has their own journey and their own timing. If you sense someone is really at the point they are ready to begin their journey, then go ahead and let them know about *Timer DIET.* But always remember that losing weight is all about *you!* So let's go through what *you* need to do—*Before You Start.*

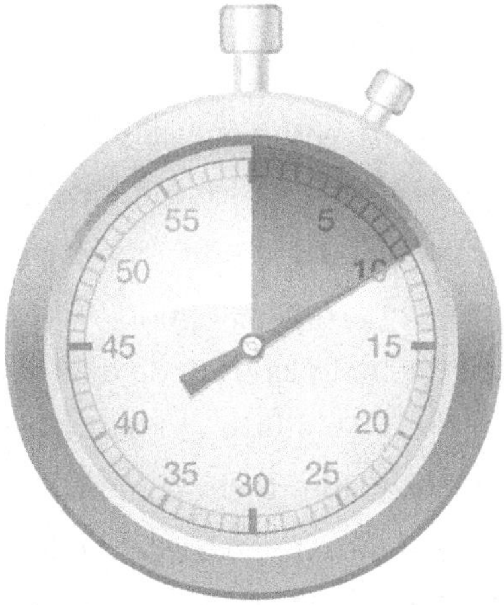

Chapter 4

Before You Start

Before you start your journey and begin to lose weight, there are a few things we need to do. We need to go through your wardrobe and see what to keep, store, toss, give away, and possibly buy. In your kitchen we need to go through the refrigerator, freezer, pantry, and spice cabinets and do the same. Next, we will create menus using foods that *you* like and will enjoy making—there may be some cooking involved once in a while; so we will go over the basics in the kitchen. We will also go over nutrients and how they are used in selecting foods for meals you make at home, restaurants you frequent, or even fast food places you may find yourself. Then we will go over all the different ways there are to track your progress and find the best method for you. Last but not least, we will work on your goals! You will pick the day to start your journey—not just any day, but *the* day that means something to *you!*

Wardrobe Makeover

Let's start with your closet. I want you to be able to wear everything that is in your closet. You may say, "That's not possible." That may not be possible right now, but it will be once we are done. This can take anywhere from 1–2 hours. You can do it in sections of time if you like, but the best plan is to do it all at once.

Remove all the clothes that you know are too small or too big for you and store them somewhere else, but close by, for future try on sessions. Sort them by size before you put them away. Do not keep them in your closet to the side; keep them completely out of sight. If you have multiple closets, you can have your current clothes in the main closet and the clothes you are not currently wearing in the other closet as long as you don't need to go into the other closet every day. If you see all of those smaller clothes every day, you are going to feel sad that you can't get into them yet, or you may be tempted to try them on when it's too early to do so

You may wonder why you are storing clothes that are *bigger* than you are now. That is because at the end of your journey we will do something great and rewarding with all the clothes that you no longer need, but more on that later, much later. Keep in mind that we are looking for clothes that fit you well. So it is possible to have different sizes in your closet during your weight loss period, because the brand sizing is different. Once you have lost your weight, we will talk about the importance of sizes. But for now, let's focus on what looks and feels great on you—right now!!

Next, go through the rest of your closet and look for clothes that need repair or have worn themselves out. Decide whether to repair them or toss them out. Go through the closet one more time, and remove anything that is unflattering on you. Look for clothes that are the wrong color or style or have been in your closet for years that you know you just won't wear. Give them away to a local charity today! This should leave you with clothes that you like, fit well, and if you went to your closet you could wear right now! If this is not the case, go back, and see what you missed. There is nothing that will adversely affect your self-esteem while losing weight more than going into your closet and trying on a pair of jeans as you are getting ready to go out the door and finding they do not fit. Don't do this to yourself! Later—once you lose a specific amount of weight, you will go to your smaller sizes and see if they fit, but it will be an event, not just some hit or miss thing as you are running out the door.

If you have gained some weight recently, and nothing seems to fit right now, you will need to buy some clothes that fit nicely and make you look good. You may say, "But I am going to lose weight. Why would I go buy clothes now?" Well, because I want you to look and feel good now—right now! Go to a discount or thrift store or buy some clothes on sale. Do not spend a lot of money (you probably will not be wearing them for long); make sure you have three pairs of pants or jeans that look good on you.

Tops are more forgiving, so what you have should be fine; but if not, get five to seven tops so you can have a little variety. Make sure you look great in them. Pick colors and styles that flatter you. Some people think that flowing tops hide flaws, but even the thinnest person will look overweight in a flowing top, so be careful that what you select actually flatters your figure. I personally like knit tops. I think they slightly hug your curves and accentuate your figure. If you aren't sure, ask someone who will not hurt your feelings if they tell you the truth. If this turns out to be the store clerk—who you may not see again—tell her you really want help picking out a certain number of items. That way she will know you are buying something and won't be inclined to tell you that *everything* looks great on you.

I love to take home all the clothes I buy and then try them on with the other clothes and shoes that I have. I do this when my makeup and hair looks somewhat decent. I start three piles—*definitely not, definitely yes,* and *maybe*? When it comes to the maybes I look at the price tag and/or try them on again and decide which of the two piles they go into. I make sure to return the items I do not feel will work for me as soon as possible.

Color, style, and fit depend a lot on personal preference, but be really sure you use your best judgment. When you drape a color next to your face, your eyes should pop or your skin glow. If you get a feeling of *uh-oh* when draping a color next to your face, it is not for you! Style is a matter of personal preference. I prefer V-necks to show off a little cleavage. Not everyone shares my sentiment. My sister gave me a long-sleeve top she didn't want and said, "Don't worry, it shows some cleavage." I laughed, but I was wondering since our styles are so different.

There is no right or wrong choice if your style is you. My only caution is that just because something is "in style" does not mean it should be *your* style. There are many things I think are so cute on the hanger, in the catalog, or on a friend, but they are just not for me. I have learned to accept this. I have preferences that are probably not other people's preferences, so I do not want to tell you exactly how to dress. Try different styles and if you change your mind, take it back. I always keep the tags on my clothes until I am ready to walk out the door in them. Keep your receipts and keep your tags on until you actually wear the item. You may be able to get store credit or a refund. This can be important if you need to buy suits or dresses and lose weight faster than you can wear the clothes you buy.

Your lingerie can make or break an outfit—it is very possible the bras and underwear you are currently wearing are not the right fit for you. Be sure your entire bra selection fits properly. Even the same brand and style of bras can fit differently. Try on each one and make sure it fits properly, and *most importantly* make sure it is comfortable and looks amazing on you! You may want to have a bra-fitting if you have never done so before, but since every style is different, it is more important to make sure *you* are comfortable and look amazing. You can find quality bras at discount stores, and most lingerie goes on sale at least twice a year. Do *not* buy bras for when you will lose weight—don't do it for any item of clothing! Just know you will probably need new bras for every 10 to 15 pounds you lose, so don't get too attached to the bras you have now! Underwear is a little different, assuming you wear it; you will want to make sure it does not create indents in your skin. Most important, make sure it is very comfortable. Lace underwear with a lot of stretch is a good choice and will also minimize lines under your garments.

Oh, the dreaded swimsuit! Always go to a store that allows you to select one size for your top and a different size for your bottom when purchasing a two-piece swimsuit. I prefer going to a store dedicated to swimsuits. They usually will have mirrors that make you look tan in the middle of winter! The other good thing is everyone else is also trying on swimsuits and you won't feel so self-conscious asking for the opinion of the sales clerk (who I have found to be very helpful in getting me the best fitting swimsuit). Again, style, color, and personal preference are all important. You may think you only want a one-piece, because that is all you have ever bought. I was surprised when I started losing weight that I really liked wearing bikinis, and I have been told I look pretty good in them! (I am sure this is in the eyes of the beholder—so be kind if you see me in one!)

My personal preference is to avoid band tops, as they flatten you out and do not provide any lift. When it comes to bottoms, the higher the cut at the thigh, the better! It will create the illusion of a longer leaner leg vs. one that cuts right at the bottom of your buttocks. Avoid skirt-type swimsuits; they add inches to your hips that you are trying so hard to lose. (Wear a matching sarong instead.) My favorite when it comes to a bikini is the triangle top and bottoms with ties on the sides. They allow you to lose weight and still look amazing. A well fitted bikini will flatter the female body. However, this is not meant to underestimate the one-piece swimsuit with ruching and other slenderizing components. They go by different names but guarantee they will make you look slimmer—and most of them do.

If you order from a catalog, know what your real cost is if you don't like something and return it. You may lose discounts on other items purchased because you returned something and you may have to pay shipping both ways. I know some clothes look amazing in a catalog, but just be sure you really like an item, since it could be a few weeks before you wear it—and then the return date, if the company allows returns, will have come and gone. Do not buy a swimsuit you are not planning on wearing soon. You are on a journey of losing weight and a swimsuit is very dependent on your size in how it fits and stays on when it is wet. Resist the temptation to buy your swimsuit in March, when the new styles come out, if you know you won't wear it until May or June—you are going to be a different size by summer!

Shoes are another thing you may not think about when you lose and gain weight. I wore a size 7 before I gained 25 plus pounds; then I was a 7.5 until I lost the weight. I bought a lot of insoles to help me keep my 7.5 shoes, since I had so many of them. You may want to wear shoes with a heel to make you look a little slimmer. Although, depending on your balance they may be harder to walk in, so use your judgment and wear the heel you're comfortable in and fits you. Avoid spending a lot of money on shoes until you have reached your maintenance weight. I bought some amazing boots when I was much heavier and now I cannot wear them, they are too loose.

Refrigerator, Freezer, Pantry, and Spice Cabinet Makeover

Cleaning out your kitchen and restocking it can feel daunting but exciting at the same time. I will try my best to help you keep the foods you have with minimal waste, yet it will be necessary to get rid of the foods you need to say good-bye to. Start with the refrigerator. Anything that is fat-free needs to go! Sugar-free foods with artificial sweeteners—in the trash! Reduced-fat foods go in the trash as well, unless the fat reduction is done naturally and without chemicals. If you cannot pronounce the ingredients or require a dictionary to figure out what the ingredients are—then it needs to go! No margarine, fat-free dressing, fat-free mayonnaise, or reduced-fat peanut butter—let it go, now! Make a list of what you are throwing out so that you can replace what you need with the real stuff.

> *Butter is as basic as it gets—salt and cream—just two basic ingredients combined together to make an amazing thing called butter. I use it every day! I think butter gets a bad reputation because people think you need to use a lot of it. Not true! I use about a teaspoon of butter when cooking my egg in the morning, and melt another teaspoon of butter for my toast. Melting your butter, before putting on your food(s) will allow you to use less, and still enjoy the taste.*

Throwing away food may be more difficult for some than others. They think of the waste, even if they are not worried about the cost. Really think about this saying, "*waste here or waist here.*" Whenever you treat your body like a garbage disposal instead of putting something in the waste bin, your waist will suffer. We do this in small ways, saying, "There are only two more bites," or in larger ways when we say, "If I don't eat this now, it will go to waste." Your body is *not* a trash can. The *Timer DIET* program emphasizes stopping as soon as you are satisfied and no later. This may mean there is one bite left or ten bites left; it really doesn't matter. While you clean out your refrigerator and deal with whether you should throw out the margarine, fat-free dressing, or sugar-free pudding, ask yourself: If I don't throw it out now, then what am I planning on doing with it? If you really can't bring yourself to throw it out, then eat *all* of it—every single bit—until there is absolutely none left before you start your weight loss program. (I obviously do *not* recommend this!)

> *We have been told time and time again to eat all of our food and to not let it go to waste because there are others who are less fortunate. I believe people's hearts are in the right place when they say this, but unfortunately, eating all of your food does NOT feed anyone else. What we need to instill upon our children (and society) is how fortunate we are and to help others who are in need. By giving of our hearts, time, and money then we can make a difference in the lives of those less fortunate and are in need—not by eating everything on our plates.*

Another important thing to do while you clean out the refrigerator is to check all of the expiration dates. You may be surprised that the pickles, mustard and ketchup expired over two-years ago! Yikes! There are different types of expiration dates. The "sell by" date is for the store; the item is not to be sold after this date—it probably has five to seven days left before it needs to be used. The "best used by date" has to do with the quality of the product diminishing after this date—it varies enormously how long a product is still consumable after this date, but just isn't at its best. The "use by" date is the last date that you should use this particular product, regardless of when you bought it. Keeping all this in mind, your sense of smell, the way the product looks, and if absolutely necessary, a tiny little taste is your best guide to know if the product isn't good enough for consumption, even if the product has not reached the date expiration. Regardless of whether the expiration date has not come and gone, my motto is: *when in doubt, throw it out!*

When you open your refrigerator you want to know that whatever you pick up is fresh, and you can eat or drink it. Assess your refrigerator at least once a week—preferably right before you go grocery shopping to avoid buying things you don't need and not buying things you didn't realize had gone bad, which could ruin your dinner plans!

Let's move onto the freezer: if you have not put the date on your frozen items and are not absolutely sure when you put them in the freezer, you will need to throw them out. That may seem wasteful, but nothing will make you want to give up on cooking more than giving yourself and others food poisoning. Remember: you want to be able to pull anything from your freezer and know that it is good. My favorite book on this subject is the *Better Homes and Gardens Cookbook*. Everyone should have a general all-purpose cookbook at their disposal. Look at the section on how long to freeze certain types of foods. If you have had something in the freezer beyond the recommended time frame or worse, you have no idea how long—then it is time to throw it away. Check everything in your freezer—even your ice cream. I used to buy a lot of the pint-size variety, and several of them had expired or had an awful frosty glaze on them. Add to your grocery list anything that you think you should keep on hand but had to throw out. You will want to keep some of your favorite meats and fish in your freezer for those "just in case" moments—remember to get into your freezer periodically and prepare your frozen foods so they do not need to throw them out.

Your pantry will also need to be looked over for items that have expired as well as items you feel are *not in your best interest* and should be removed. Somehow, right before deciding to lose weight, I bought a case of individual microwavable macaroni and cheese. I am not saying that you cannot have macaroni and cheese; you can, but freshly made would be better than microwavable and I certainly did not need a *case.* I gave it a way to the food pantry at my local grocery store, which if you have any non-perishable items that you want to give away is your best option.

Last but not least, your spice cabinet needs a once-over as well. Look for spices that have expired, and toss them (*you do not need to toss your decorative spices—I never use them they just look nice on the counter*). Spices can actually go rancid and make a wonderful dish a disaster. It is better to throw a spice out now than to find out after the fact a bad spice just ruined an afternoon of cooking a certain dish for a special occasion.

Look for spices that you really don't like. You tried them once or twice, and they just were not your thing. When you are cooking you want to know that any spice you select you will enjoy. Toss them now or set them aside, and wait for them to expire. (I know someone wants to do that!) Also, look to see that you have enough of your favorite spices. The last thing you want is to be cooking dinner and find you have only one shake left of your favorite garlic salt or nothing to refill your black pepper grinder. Check everything, as your spices are going to make your meals amazing!

Kitchen Makeover

The most important item to have in any kitchen, whether you are a novice or seasoned chef, is a fire extinguisher that is especially made for the kitchen. This is not because I believe you will start a fire! But, it can happen, even to the most experienced. I have yet to need to use the fire extinguisher—I have two of them. Have one in the kitchen and I keep another one in the closest room to the kitchen either in a bathroom or laundry room. (You may get a discount on your homeowners insurance or your homeowners insurance may say that you must already have at least one.) Check the expiration date of the extinguishers and put the date to replace them in your calendar. If you have never used one before, read over the directions at least once, so you are not reading them for the first time if you need to use it. Not all fires require a fire extinguisher, but ***never*** put water on a kitchen fire!

I like to have three of everything that is important enough to use almost every day—one is in the dishwasher, one is being used, and one will need to be used. In some cases, one may be ready to break!

Egg slicer	1 qt. Saucier w/spout	Small Cutting Boards
Paring Knives	Spatulas	Tongs—short and long
6 oz. Custard Cups	Glass Measuring Cups	Dry Measuring Cups/Spoons

A knife set that sits on the cabinet and includes steak knives and scissors with teeth in the center for opening things will be invaluable when you are cooking. Knife blocks are attractive, organized, and you always know where they are. While I keep extra knives in the drawer, my go-to knives are on the counter. I use them every day! It is not necessary to spend a lot of money for good quality, but check out reviews if you are not sure what brand to get for the best value.

Pepper grinders are a great asset to any kitchen. I love my pepper grinder, but I have tried many that do not provide me with variable grinds or the coarsest grind is too fine for me. If you are able to try them out, you should; at the very least read the packaging very carefully and compare to others to see what type of grinds it will do. I do not have a salt grinder as of now, but I have thought about getting one mostly to have one on the counter. I love my kosher salt and right now I keep it in the original box.

Pots and pans are a must in any kitchen. You need to have at least one pan that you can cook breakfast in—a 10-Inch skillet is a good size to have. I also like to have an 8-Inch skillet just in case the mood strikes for an omelet. You will also need an 8-Quart stock pot with a cover for boiling water. A 4-Quart sauté pan and 2-Quart saucepan with matching covers will complete your basic set of pots and pans. These can be bought together as a set or individually, it does not matter. The prices can vary from the modest to the expensive. If you want to get the best that you can for the least amount of money, check out discount and thrift stores, and online retailers. It is not necessary to make an enormous investment in your pots and pans.

Steamers are a must and come in several styles. There are stainless steel collapsible steamers that fit into a pot or pan. Rice cookers can have an extra attachment that makes them into a steamer. A steamer that stands on its own is my preference and is relatively inexpensive and easy to clean, which is important considering you will probably use it several times per week. I really did not get into steaming vegetables until I decided to lose weight. I either bought canned vegetables, ate them raw, or more than likely I avoided vegetables unless they were in a salad. Now that I own a steamer, I love cooked vegetables.

Another must-have is an indoor grill. It is fine if you want to cook outdoors on the grill, but let's face it—no matter where you live, there will be days, if not months, when cooking outside just isn't going to happen. ***Never*** bring an outdoor grill inside your home. The manual will tell you this, but just in case you lost the manual, it is dangerous, so never do it. There are several indoor grills on the market; some are relatively inexpensive. Search online and get reviews. There are smaller ones if you prefer and are grilling for one or two people. You can also bake your meals—and we will discuss how to do that—but the indoor grill is my mainstay when it comes to steak, chicken, and many fish entrées.

I love Tupperware! I used to sell it back in my college days, and I have a lot of it. I know there are other products that are similar, but for me, there is only Tupperware. Having said that, your leftovers need to be kept fresh—so choose containers that are airtight and watertight. You will also want a 6-Cup bowl with a watertight lid for shaking up individual salads, which will insure the dressing gets all over the lettuce. While I recommend having a variety of disposable containers for houseguests you want to send home with leftovers, it is best to invest in reusable containers for yourself. Some of you may not believe in eating leftovers. I promise they can be as good as the original. In some cases, dishes are even better the next day! I will give you hints on how to spice them up by adding a little something to them and how to reheat them so they are not over-cooked. You may decide you like leftovers so much that you start intentionally cooking more food, so you have leftovers—saving you time on cooking!

Special containers and bags may keep your foods fresh longer. There are different kinds and different uses. There are bags designed to prolong the life for produce items such as lettuce, tomatoes, broccoli, carrots, cauliflower, and green onions. There are also containers that are meant for berries, pineapple, watermelon, and cantaloupe. An onion saver may also be beneficial in keeping the onion smell away from other foods in your refrigerator. If your food is not staying fresh as long as you need it to, check out what options are available. Food storage bags with a suction feature for bacon, steak and chicken are great when you do not use the entire package at one meal. Be sure your kitchen has a felt-tip pen/marker and removable garage sale labels so you can write the date on them. Everything that is taken out of its original container or does not already have a date, like fresh produce, needs a date on it.

If you are able to write directly on the bag, this is preferable, but if not, then use the labels. This will save you time, money, and aggravation!

New dishes can change your dynamic with food. If you are even remotely thinking about getting new dishes, go ahead and do it now. It can be a great way to say, "We are starting something new!". When deciding on what dishes to get think about the size of each dish. Lunch plates or bread plates are the perfect size for many meals or mini-meals. You want dishes that make your food look like your plate is not too cramped and not too empty. Also, if your current dishes are not microwaveable (for reheating) or dishwasher safe, you may want to get dishes that are, since you will doing a lot more cooking—and really you will be doing a lot more eating.

If you are used to eating out of containers, that is going to change. Every meal is going to be an enjoyable presentation on a plate that is the appropriate size for what you are eating. You will probably run the dishwasher at least once a day. If you are used to going out to eat all the time, you will actually save time and money. That is not to say that you can't eat out for social or entertainment value, but you won't need to go to a restaurant, because you would otherwise starve—I promise, it will be easy!

Cooking

It is very important to know the basics of cooking—not only so that you have more fresh food options that you can create into wonderful meals for you and your family, but also because without the basics of cooking, you will end up buying premade foods that most likely will be processed. This can impede your weight loss. Your cooking skills do not need to be fancy. Of course—you will want to know how to use knives to chop, dice, and slice without cutting yourself!! And, you will also need to know the difference between stir vs. fold; sauté vs. cook;

and bake vs. broil. *Always* check your oven before turning it on to make sure nothing is in it that you forgot or did not know about! The best thing to do if you have never grilled a steak or baked a potato is to have a trusted friend or family member show you the basics. You could take a class if you really feel you need to. But before you do look at *Appendix B—Cooking,* this appendix may help you learn the basics. My trusted cookbook, *Better Homes and Gardens,* can also give you a lot of guidance on what you need to know in the kitchen as well. If you have never seen a general all-purpose cookbook, now is a great time to get one and just skim through it so you know all that it has to offer, whether you are a beginner or already know your way around the kitchen.

If you do not know how to cook, when you go through the menu ideas, stick to those that do not require much cooking until you get yourself acclimated in the kitchen. Once you do and realize the power this knowledge will give you, you will be very glad you learned how to cook.

Nutrients

Most people think they know what nutrients are in most foods but in many cases are wrong. Here is a short quiz: for each food item, pick *a, b,* or *c* as the primary selected nutrient for each item, and then rank the other two in order of significance.

a) Dietary Fat b) Carbohydrates c) Protein

1. Vanilla ice cream
2. Eggs
3. Steak tenderloin
4. Fresh strawberries
5. Whole milk
6. Potato chips
7. Beef jerky
8. Salsa
9. Cheddar cheese
10. Fresh broccoli

The answers are in *Appendix C—Menus and Restaurant Guide.* I included the estimated grams for each selected nutrient per the National Agricultural Library. How did you do? Are you surprised? My goal here is to help you realize you may not know what you think you know about nutrient ratios of popular foods.

It is not so much that there are *bad* foods as much as there are bad combinations of foods. Let's say you want to enjoy a piece of birthday cake. You can, but before you eat the cake, you should eat something with protein to counteract the carbohydrates and dietary fat in the cake and frosting. A piece of chicken or grilled fish with a green vegetable would be a good entrée to have when you know you will be having dessert. It is really all about counteracting each category. For example; if what you *want* is mostly dietary fat, you will need to add some carbohydrates and protein to what you *want.* Most importantly you do not want to overeat! It just takes a little practice.

Recommended percentages of dietary fat, protein, and carbohydrates vary with different programs or diets, and can become cumbersome to keep your meals within specific percentages. The *Timer DIET* guideline is to ideally include all three at each meal or mini-meal and have the ratio of grams be somewhat close to each other, but necessarily equal. For example, if I want a can of chili with beans and the carbohydrates are four times the dietary fat and twice the protein I know I need to add more dietary fat and a little more protein—therefore I would add shredded cheddar cheese. I have counteracted the imbalance and I am good to go!! (See—*How to Read a Label*—below.)

These days' restaurants provide the food values for most of their menu items. Take advantage of this information. The Internet is the best place to locate the nutritional values. If there are certain restaurants you normally go to, check them out online. I bet you will be surprised to find out there are a lot of healthy menu items that are already well-balanced; although the portions may be more than you will want to eat in one sitting. Which brings up one of my favorite things about going out to eat and that is—embracing leftovers! I can get anywhere from one to three more meals out of leftovers—most restaurants serve too much food to be eaten at one sitting.

Fast food should be on an as-needed basis. Maybe you are out shopping and didn't bring a snack or time doesn't permit sitting down to eat. Every fast food restaurant has something that is well-balanced and won't get you off track—you may need to throw some of it away. More than likely, leftovers will not be good from a fast food place. Food values are constantly changing as well as what menu items are offered, so check your favorite fast food restaurants website before you start your weight loss program so you can make wise choices on the spot! My favorite quick eat is little chicken pieces that are fried with no sauce at all. I omit the sauce for several reasons: there is usually a lot of sugar in sauces; I am also in a hurry and it is easier to eat while I drive without sauce; and I also really like the taste without the sauce.

When it comes to fast food restaurants, calories are not the be all and end all in your food choices, but they must be considered in this world of options that can give you an entire day's worth of calories and not much to show for them. When you check out the grams of dietary fat, protein, and carbohydrates, go ahead and look at the calories, and make your choice wisely. Not all options are created equal, but there is almost always something on the menu that will work, even if it means eating a smaller portion of it to tide you over until you get home.

Grocery Shopping and Menu Creating

Before you go grocery shopping, you will want to make a list of the items you want to buy. This is more than just being organized; it is about making sure that you buy only items you have put some thought into. Make sure everything you buy has a purpose. When you make a purchase, know when and how you are going to eat it. What will it go with? Knowing your entire meal plan is very important. If you buy cottage cheese but no fruit, you will not have a complete meal. The same thought process is needed for fruits and vegetables. What do you plan to eat with them? Fruits and vegetables are mostly carbohydrates, so the best pairing for fruits are cheeses, and vegetables go great with meat, poultry, or seafood.

The main thing you want to do before you go grocery shopping is to make your menus. They don't need to be elaborate, and they can be done by categories. For example, on Monday for dinner, you could have steak and a vegetable with a salad to start. It is not necessary at the time of creating your menu to know what kind of steak or which vegetable. When you buy eggs, do you already know what you are going to eat with them? My suggestion is Canadian or regular bacon. Smoked salmon is also good with hard-boiled eggs. Don't forget some grains, maybe toast or a *little* oatmeal (¼ cup or less) if you prefer, for breakfast. The point of making your menu plans is that you have already created items that go together that you like. This makes it easier to create your grocery list and avoid buying foods that may go to waste. If you are responsible for others, hopefully they will like the food combinations as well. You may want to include them with the menu planning; it can be a great learning tool.

Make your menus like a restaurant: breakfast, lunch/dinner, and smaller mini-meals for in-between times. When you create your menus, be sure to have a variety of ideas that take different amounts of time to make and eat. I made menus that consisted of items that took one minute to make, like tomatoes with a hard-boiled egg. While others were more elaborate, like taco night or a steak dinner with all the trimmings that takes up to 30 minutes to prepare. In *Chapter 5—How to Do It!* there are detailed sample menus based on lifestyle and in

Appendix C—Menus and Restaurant Guide there are ideas to help you create your own menus that you and your family and friends will love!

Checklist to go over before grocery shopping:

- » ***Always check the expiration date.*** If you can't find the expiration date, don't buy it. Make sure you know todays date. I have to admit, I have looked at an expiration date not realizing I did not know what day it was. I got home only to realize then I only had one day to eat it.
- » ***Read labels to make sure that you understand the ingredients without a medical dictionary.*** Do not buy anything with artificial sweeteners or fat reducers. With a little practice, you should be able to do a detailed analysis of a label in less than 15 seconds! (See below)
- » ***Do not pay any attention to the front packaging!*** It may say *nutritious, healthy,* or *smart,* but all of these sayings are fluff. Marketing companies work very hard to come up with words that sound healthy but really do not mean anything on their own—like *wholesome, lite,* or *only 100 calories*. If the packaging is trying to sell you, there is probably a reason. Vegetables do not try to sell you, do they? They are just hanging out in the produce section with a price per pound—no frills, no fuss!
- » ***Stick to your list, but if you find something you need or want, go ahead and get it if it makes sense to your overall menu plan.*** Let's face it—you can't think of everything. Sometimes you see something and think; *I could really make that work for dinner this week*. So why not get it?
- » ***Have your meal plans ready and with you.*** In *Appendix A—Grocery Lists* and *Appendix C—Menus and Restaurant Guide* you will find suggestions based on type of meal and length of

time needed to prepare. Before you start, you will need to create your own menus based on foods you already like or may want to incorporate into the new lifestyle you are creating.

How to read a food label

Food labels have several important pieces of information. The focus will be on grams not calories. Most diets will ask you to calculate how many calories per gram in order to know the ratios they recommend (there are 9 grams per calorie for dietary fat and 4 grams per calorie for protein and carbohydrates). This calculation can be cumbersome and difficult when you are grocery shopping and want to get through the store without constantly going to your calculator. Since the *Timer DIET* is based on grams which are already included on the label this should make for easier label reading. Let's look at the numerous pieces of information included on a food label that are of importance and those that are merely anecdotal—starting from top to bottom:

- » Serving Size—only eat what you feel comfortable eating—therefore, anecdotal
- » Calories—only for comparison to the serving size—again, anecdotal
- » Total Fat grams—*no less than half and no more than double* protein or carbohydrates
- » Trans Fat—ideally should be zero or less than one percent
- » Sodium—a meal should be no more than 25 percent of the daily recommendation
- » Total Carbohydrate—*no less than half and no more than double* the dietary fat or protein
- » Protein—*no less than half and no more than double* the dietary fat or carbohydrates

This portion of the label should take about 15 seconds to process, based on multiplying and dividing by two for your comparisons of the dietary fat, protein, and carbohydrates. Reading the ingredients may take a little longer to process. The good thing is that once you have established which foods you feel you should eat you do not need to continually read the labels.

Ingredients are important to look at when you are grocery shopping. This all may seem overwhelming at first but I promise it will get easier. The ingredients are listed in order from the most to the least. However, they do not tell you the percentage. So the first ingredient could be anywhere from 1% (if there were over 100 ingredients) or 100% if there was only one ingredient. The reality is you do not know how much of each ingredient is in a food only the order. It is a good bet that you are primarily eating the first two to three ingredients. This may be surprising when you look at the label. You will need to decide if you are willing to eat something that has as its first ingredient something which you do not even feel should be in the product. Mayonnaise comes to mind, the first ingredient is soybean oil. I like mayonnaise and have no plans to stop eating it. I also do not eat it every day. (Since I take thyroid medicine I need to limit my soy intake.) But, I was surprised when I looked at the label. Most of your foods will be fresh foods, so there will not be a label to read. Understanding the foods you like to eat on a routine basis will be necessary.

Explaining the ratios

As you may notice the ratios of dietary fat, protein, and carbohydrates can vary significantly. This is by design. Not every meal or mini-meal is the same and to try to make them so creates significant limitations to your time and options. What I specifically wanted to avoid when deciding to lose weight. Most all meals or mini-meals will be well-balanced—that is the goal. Perhaps there may be more dietary fat for breakfast and less for lunch. I did not want to have to continually concern myself with the numbers, but yet I wanted some guidelines to help me. I created the following saying, "No less than half, no more than double." So when I look at a label, I can easily see if I need to add something to balance it out a little more.

I am sure your first objection to this is, *how I can possibly promote double the dietary fat of protein and carbohydrates—Almonds!* Who has not had a diet book recommend some almonds as a snack? They are great! But, the ratios of one ounce of almonds are approximately as follows:

	Percentages Based on grams	Percentages Based on calories
Dietary Fat	55%	74%
Carbohydrates	22.5%	13%
Protein	22.5%	13%

As you can see the ratio of dietary fat is a little more than double that of the carbohydrates and protein based on grams. Would I eat almonds or foods with this ratio all day—No! But, I also would not eliminate them either.

Perhaps another concern is getting too much protein—Cottage Cheese 4%-milkfat! The ratios of half a cup of cottage cheese containing 4%-milkfat is approximately:

	Percentages Based on grams	Percentages Based on calories
Dietary Fat	23%	40%
Carbohydrates	18%	14%
Protein	59%	46%

I may add a little fruit to the cottage cheese to increase the ratio of carbohydrates, thus reducing the protein and dietary fat ratios as well or I may not.

This is about as detailed into numbers as we will get. Do not get hung up on the ratios; use them as guidelines when deciding what to eat and how to make your menus. If something is a little more than double or a little less than half, so be it. See how you feel and if necessary compensate with a food that has the nutrient that was minimal to offset the imbalance. This part is not meant to be difficult; it is a way to provide you with guidance. The main focus is to not overeat and eating a well-balanced diet is going to help you with this goal.

Are you hungry?

Let's assume you have your grocery list and are ready to go grocery shopping. Stop for a second and make sure you are not hungry. How long has it been since you last ate? If has been more than a couple of hours, take a moment and eat a little something before you go. If it has not been more than two hours, grab a cheese stick and a bottle of water, and take it along with you so that if you get hungry or thirsty while you are there, you will have something to tide you over. If you are already at the grocery store and you forgot to think about whether you were hungry or you did think about it and once you got there all of a sudden you decide now you are hungry, don't worry! Go to the deli counter (not the bakery!). The deli counter people will give you samples of the meats and cheeses in their deli case. Usually a slice or two of either should make you feel much better. If you completely underestimated your hunger or just do not feel comfortable asking for a sample, go ahead and make your deli purchases first, and then eat some of what you have bought.

You may think it is no big deal to be hungry while you are grocery shopping; besides you have a list. But, if you are not thinking properly because you are hungry, something is not going to go as planned when you are at the grocery store. Maybe you decide not to follow your list, forget to check expiration dates, or don't bother to look at a label to see that a certain goat cheese has 7 g of carbohydrates while another type has only 2 g. You do not want to be hurried and thinking about other things. Most importantly you do not want to be thinking—*when can I get out of here and eat?*

You are almost ready

Now, you are ready to go grocery shopping—*almost*: you may have heard the perimeter of the grocery store has all the fresh foods and the aisles have the canned, frozen, and boxed items, and to stay in the perimeter. But, I think every kitchen needs to have some of all the above. You don't want to go grocery shopping every other day, and you don't want so much fresh food that it goes bad before you get a chance to eat it all. Go ahead and buy some canned, boxed, and especially frozen foods for times when you just don't have time to cook on a grill or steam vegetables—just don't make them your main source of nutrition.

Another issue that seems to be more commonplace these days is food recalls. They can be fresh, frozen, boxed, or canned food recalls—nothing is immune. Do you have a reliable source to know if there are food recalls you need to concern yourself with? I normally watch the local news, but if you are not a frequent news watcher, you will want to set up some breaking news alerts to know of any food recalls in your local area.

You are at the grocery store—finally!

Avoid aisles with items not on your shopping list, like soda, potato chips, and cookies, if at all possible (it is not a coincidence that the laundry detergent is on the same aisle as the cookies and candy)—look the other way!! Don't worry; you won't even miss the cookie and candy aisle once you start eating foods that you love. If you do want dessert, make something from scratch! Make a batch of brownies, a dozen cookies, or a delicious cake. I mean get out the flour and the sugar and baking powder—you want your desserts to be enjoyable but not easy to get to. This is why you don't want to keep a bag of cookies or chips in the pantry; they are too easy to get into and eat without even thinking about it.

> *Grocery shopping close to dinnertime may be problematic—the last thing you may want to do is come home and cook, I get it!! Pick up something like a premade roasted chicken from the deli counter and add a salad, so you can feed you and everyone else as soon as you get home from the grocery store. I do this for me and my dog Princie—he loves it!!*

Coming home from the grocery store

When you do come home from grocery shopping it is important to take a little extra time and make sure you have everything organized in the refrigerator and freezer so you can easily see it and know that it is fresh for your meals. You do not want to buy something at the grocery store only to find out that you really had it but it was hidden. That wastes time and money and will make you none too happy! Be sure your fruits and vegetables are in food containers that will maximize their freshness. Decide now if there are some foods that should be frozen and then thawed when ready to eat. If any of your fruits need to be cut in order to be eaten, now is the time to do it—pineapple and watermelon come to mind—your produce department *may* do this for you, if you ask.

Be sure to date everything, which is not either already dated or is removed from its original container, with the current date so you remember when it was purchased. For instance, if I were to buy tomatoes, lettuce, onions, strawberries, bananas, steak, and swordfish: I would put the tomatoes and lettuce into individual bags writing the full date on the bags. The onion would go in an onion saver and with the felt-tip marker write the date purchased on the cover (it *should* wipe off). The strawberries would go into containers meant to keep them fresh longer. Write the purchase date on the *removable labels you have in your kitchen*. Just remember to take it off before putting it in the dishwasher. The bananas go on a banana hanger where I can see how they are doing.

How I package the steak would depend on whether I was ready to freeze it or just refrigerate it. If I were ready to freeze the steak I would put each fillet into individual freezer bags—the kind that allow me to remove the air; I would write the date I was putting the steak in the freezer on the bag. The reason for freezing them individually is so they will thaw correctly in cold water when I am ready to use them. However, if I were just refrigerating the steak I would keep them in the original container until I was ready to eat them; then if I did not cook all of the steak I would put the remaining fillets in a bag meant just for the refrigerator—also the kind that allows me to remove the air; the date I would write on the package is the date purchased with an arrow writing the use by date from the original packaging. This way I will know when I must either eat or freeze the steak at a glance. The swordfish is most likely already frozen at the grocery store, so I would put it in different type of freezer bag (not necessarily the kind with the air removal feature, since the swordfish should already be packaged appropriately) with the purchase date written on the bag so I can see it easier.

With a little bit of planning and organization, you will be able to go grocery shopping and stay within your budget, since you won't be wasting food by having them go bad on you—or worse yet, buying them when they are already expired!

Journals

Journals give you valuable information in your weight loss journey. Everyone is different: there are not two people who need the exact same foods, in the exact same quantity, at the exact same time of day to lose weight or to feel good for that matter. This is why tracking what *you* eat and how *you* exercise is so important; it helps you learn about *you*. At *www.timerdiet.com,*there are nutrition and exercise journals you can print out. There is also an Android and Apple app, *Timer DIET.* This App is designed for you to track your daily food entries and can also be accessed through the website. I am a little old school, and personally like paper just so I can write notes all over. Words of encouragement, caution, or suggestions help me do better in meeting my goals. Phrases like *You did it!*, *OMG*, or *workout a little more*, give me much needed introspection or affirmation. There are words of encouragement or motivation included in the App and website if you choose to use them as your journal. The exercise portion of your journal is just as important. Tracking your fitness progress will give you a lot of insight as to what it takes to stay on track and meet your weight loss goals. For now we will focus on the nutrition journal.

You will want to be comfortable with your method of tracking meals and exercise *before* you start your weight loss program. Try all the possible ways to keep track of your progress—let me show you why this is important.

Print out a *Nutrition Journal* from *www.timerdiet.com/journal* (you can also write on a piece of paper, if you prefer). Write down what you remember eating and approximately when you ate for the last two days. It doesn't have to be a perfect memory. There is no need to write how much you ate. My guess is that it was hard to remember everything you ate over the last two days, let alone when you ate. If that was too easy: What did you eat for lunch three weeks ago on Tuesday and what time did you eat?

This is the main reason for writing down what and when you ate—it is impossible to remember and the information you will glean from your journals will be invaluable in your journey.

Let's do a couple of exercises to prepare you for keeping track of your daily progress:

For the next week or so, practice tracking what you eat and when you eat it. It is not important *what* you eat or *when* you eat it! We are only looking for which method works best for you *before it matters!* You can try one method each day or at different times of the day—whatever you want. Evaluate your options so you have one main method and two backup methods for when you are away from your main one. Here are some options I have for you to try:

Main Methods

- Nutrition Journal printouts from *www.timerdiet.com/journal*
  - *Kept in a 3-ring binder*
  - *Kept in a specialty binder*
  - *Kept with just a ring or a binder clip*
- Website-Member Portal at *www.timerdiet.com/login*
- *Timer DIET* App either Android or Apple—also a backup method

Backup Methods

- *Timer DIET* App either Android or Apple—also a main method
- Texting to yourself (text to your own cell—this is handy if you are using the written journal but are out and about—this will automatically time stamp your entry if done when eating)
- E-mailing yourself (same concept as texting)

» Keep a small writing tablet in your purse (if you want to forgo all technology—this would be used with the printed journals—for while you are on the go)

Finding the method of tracking your progress *before you start* will be crucial to your success, so do not skip this step. It will take a little practice to get used to doing but once it becomes a part of your routine, it will be easy!

Bad Habits and Vices

In the late '70s I worked as a grocery store clerk. A young woman in her mid-twenties, a little heavy, not excessively so, asked me what brand of cigarettes she should buy. At the time I smoked, so I agreed to help her decide. (I quit smoking decades ago!) I asked her what she was used to smoking, and that is when she informed me that she did not smoke—*yet*—but was going to take it up so she could lose weight! I obviously discouraged her. *Never* take up a bad habit to lose weight! It is not necessary and then you are going to need to give up the new bad habit. But most of all, you will associate the bad habit with why you lost weight, so when you try to give it up, you most likely will gain back the weight.

Diet pills and abuse of prescription drugs is another no-no! I personally do not think any pill or herb is needed to lose weight; you have the power to lose the weight yourself. What happens if you do end up losing weight using a pill? You can't stay on the pill forever, and you now have to give credit to the pill and not your own abilities. It is a double whammy; you can't take credit for losing the weight, and when you stop taking the pill, you are probably going to gain the weight back, even if only because you now have associated your weight loss to the pill.

A chiropractor begged me to try these little balls behind the ears. He wanted me to try them so badly that when I continued my resistance, he said he would put them on my ears for free. Even though I had already been losing weight—about half of my final goal—and I met every weekly goal thus far; I gave in and let him put them behind my ears. I wore them for three days and took them off. I told my chiropractor they just didn't work for me. What really happened was that I started to feel nauseous—not getting sick nauseous—more like something didn't feel right nauseous. At this point in my journey, I had no idea that a weight loss book was in my future. I just felt that I had worked so hard to lose the weight on my own so far; that there was no way I was going to give some little balls credit for reaching my final goal. So I took them off—never to be seen again.

Mints and chewing gum are other habits that may not bode well for you in your weight loss journey. I personally believe that chewing should be for when you are eating, which would rule out chewing gum (unless just to freshen your breath quickly for a face-to-face meeting). I also don't believe in sugar substitutes which most gum has in it. Also, if you take up chewing gum as a way to avoid eating, you may affect your appetite in a bad way. You want your body to let you know when it is really hungry, and chewing gum can keep this feeling from being triggered in a timely manner. Mints, even if they don't have sugar substitutes, still do not serve your weight loss purpose and can also cause the feeling of hunger to be dismissed. As a possible alternative, if you want to brush your teeth with a very soft toothbrush and super-small amount of gentle toothpaste after every meal, then I guess that is fine. Doing this may keep you from wanting to eat for a little while if that seems to be a problem you are dealing with. Make sure your dentist feels this is okay for you to do.

How Did I Get Here?

Take the time, before you start your weight loss journey, to write in your journal how you got to where you are now in having gained the weight. Did something specific happen in your life that caused a lot of stress or took up your time? Was there a specific point when you recall just saying, "I don't care anymore"? Don't filter yourself. Write down as much as you can recall. Sometimes days turn into decades and the details can get lost. Try to write down at least three things you feel contributed to your weight gain. If you can't, that's fine—or perhaps unfortunately, you have been overweight since your childhood. If so, write down what you may have done as an adult that did not help you in your weight loss journeys in the past.

This introspection may be very valuable and you may want to look back on what you have written, especially when you encounter slow progress, to see if you are engaging in any of these old habits again. For now, just keep them in your journal, and if you are lucky, you will not need to refer to them again. Hopefully, writing them down will release them from your past.

Loving Life, Stress, and Giving

During each day, what do you think about? What do you look forward to? Are there people or pets that you can look to for love and companionship? I hope so. If not, I would see about getting this part of your life in order as soon as possible. Life is short; so love the people who love you. Whether two-legged or four-legged—enjoy their company. It surprises me how often we have people in our lives whom we don't love to be with. This can be a great source of stress, and stress can make it hard to lose weight. I am not saying to get rid of all the people in your life who cause you stress; you would be alone. But if you are not enjoying them as much as you wish you could, do something about it; make a conscious effort to appreciate them—remembering why you wanted them in your life in the first place. You may be surprised how doing just this one little thing makes your time with them more pleasant and less stressful.

Stress is not avoidable and sometimes in life it is necessary to get you going. But, if you find you are easily stressed (most of us are) then make a list ahead of time of things that you can do to relieve stress immediately, routinely, and long-term.

Examples of stress relief ideas:

- Immediate Stress Relief
  - Aromatherapy
  - Close eyes for a few minutes and breathe deeply
  - Listen to a specific song or some music

- Routine Activities to Reduce Stress
  - Schedule some play-time (fun) each week
  - Workout aerobically for 30 minutes daily
  - Spend time with friends at least once a week

- Long-term ways to Reduce Stress
  - Have mini-vacations planned for a few times a year
  - Plan on a visit with the grandkids or nieces and nephews
  - Finish a big project and celebrate it!

Giving is another stress reducer. We can give to those we know, and we can give to those we don't know: either with our time or our money. If you don't already give to those you don't know, I highly recommend it. You can start out very small if your budget doesn't allow for much. Most charities will accept just a few dollars and be very grateful for your donation. I don't know how to explain it *yet*, but giving to others, when it does not personally benefit you, is a great feeling!

Giving Up One Food

Before we go over your goals think of one food you could give up only while you are losing weight. It should be something that is not intrinsically or potentially harmful if you add it back to your diet. (Artificial sweeteners or high-sugar drinks are not what we are talking about.) It also should not be something general, like sugar or chocolate. I gave up french fries, since I knew that they are easy to eat a lot of without thinking, and I also knew that I was not planning on going without them forever. They also were not something that I ate all of the time already, so I would not feel giving up french fries is *why* I reached my goals. I wanted a symbol of reaching my goal and transitioning over to maintenance—for me that was french fries. Hopefully you already had a food in mind to give up only for the time you were losing weight. If not, think of one now.

Goal Setting

You have a few goals and time tables to work out before you get started. You will need to decide when to start, how much to lose, what dress size you want to be in, when you want to achieve your goal by, how much per week you plan to lose, and at what weight you want to stay. We will go into revising your goals more in *Chapter 9—Now that You Have Lost the Weight.*

Be sure that you are conservative in your weight loss goals and feel confident you can and should weigh the amount that you have chosen. Some people mistakenly think they should get back to the weight they were in high school or on their wedding day. These historical frames of reference, while they may seem reasonable, probably are not. Most adults will re-characterize their body as they get older. We change our muscle mass and fat composition. If I weighed now what I weighed in high school, I am sure I would look very sickly. I didn't look sickly at the time: I was much younger and slender, with less padding on my hips and breasts, and basically no thigh fat to speak of.

Always keep in mind *you* are making your weight loss goals and no one else: When I was in my early 20's I interviewed for an airline. I weighed in at 108 pounds for my second interview. I was told *if* they hired me, I would be on probation until I lost three pounds and must maintain my *mandated* reduced weight while employed. Even at the time I did not feel losing weight would be healthy for me (mentally or physically) and I did not want to let someone else tell me what I should weigh. As you can imagine, I did not fare so well in the final interview.

You also don't want to lose so much weight that you cannot afford a sudden weight loss due to illness or some other unexpected event. A good rule of thumb is to be sure you can afford to lose another five pounds if you were to become ill. If you feel that you can decide on a weight that is truly in your best interest—great, go for it. But if not, focus on the smaller goals, and reevaluate your long-term goal as you see how you look and feel as you lose weight. Be sure to decide ahead of time when you will reevaluate your goals if you do not know for sure how much you want to weigh when you are done with your weight loss journey.

> *In the end it is all about how much* **you** *want to weigh—not your friends, family, or personal trainer. You need to feel comfortable and sexy with you! If you are in a committed sexual relationship, do not miss opportunities to have sex with your partner, especially if you do not feel sexy. Feeling sexy will be easier when you are having more sex, and feeling*

sexy will cause you to not want to overeat. Lest you single people feel that this is something that requires a partner—it is not! Never say to yourself or anyone else that you are not sexy. You may have excess weight, but that does not mean you are not sexy.

Let's get started on setting your goals! There may be something going on in your life which makes you more interested in the end date, for others it may be the start date—either could be a birthday, holiday, or some other event. While others really don't care about what day they start *or* stop; they just want to be a size 6—period!

Let's go through the thought process for my goals: I mostly wanted to be in a size 6 by summer (a little vague at first). The start date I wanted to be soon, but at the same time I wanted to have a start date that I would remember. The 1st of the month I thought would be easy to remember someday in the future, after time had passed and I was reminiscing. As luck would have it, my goal-setting session began mid-February of 2009, and the 1st of March was coming up. I knew I would be busy working during the month of March, so I figured if I could keep up a workout schedule during the busiest time of the year, I could do it anytime! Okay, so I had a start date: March 1st and I wanted to weigh 130 (which I thought would be a size 6 for me). I was currently about 150 pounds so that was 20 pounds I needed to lose. I thought one pound a week seemed pretty reasonable, so I did the math and saw that I would reach my goal mid-July a little later than I had hoped—I had started to think my birthday was a good date to reach my goal by. My birthday however, is in late June, I decided I could reach my goal in 17 weeks instead of 20 weeks (I went on faith that there must be a few weeks where I would lose a little more than one pound) and therefore, reach my goal by my 47th birthday. Now I was excited, I had a goal, it was tied into my birthday and it was starting soon! Everything seemed very doable (although at this point I still had no idea *what* I was going to do to lose weight—but I did not let that bother me—my only focus was my goals).

Here are the goals I made that day, back in February 2009:

- » *Start on March 1, 2009*
- » *Goal date on June 23, 2009 – my birthday*
- » *Stop and reassess weight goals on June 24, 2009*
- » *Lose 20 pounds – weigh 130 pounds*
- » *Be a dress size 6*

Now on to short-term or mini-goals: Every Friday would be my goal day, and every week the goal would be one pound. I picked Friday, since I didn't want to focus my weekends on my goals. My weekends were actually filled with relief that I had met one more week's goal. I also kept my goals as a positive number rather than as the amount I needed to lose. I think the focus on my goal weight helped me a lot. Let's say I start at 150.2 pounds my goal for the next Friday would be 149.2 pounds, so every morning I would get on the scale I would say to myself, "149.2, 149.2, 149.2" until I was actually 149.2 pounds by my goal date. Sometimes reaching a weekly goal took a few days, and sometimes it took all seven days. But once I reached it during the week, it counted.

Let me explain: If I was down to 145.4 pounds on a Friday, and I set my next week's goal at 144.4 pounds, if by Wednesday I was already at 144.4 pounds, I would have already met my goal for the week! It didn't matter that on Friday, I was at 144.6 pounds; this did not negate the fact that I reached my goal for the week. I was already on to a new goal, and that was 143.4 by the next Friday. Now let's look at a different scenario.

Next scenario: If on Friday, I weighed 144.2 pounds and I made my goal for next Friday—143.2 pounds, but by the time Friday came, I actually weighed 142.8 pounds Awesome! I met my goal, and the next Friday's goal would be 141.8 pounds—one pound less than the lowest amount on Friday *or* the goal weight reached for the week.

Last scenario: I set my goal for 147.8 pounds to be reached by Friday, at one point during the week I weighed 147.2 pounds, and then by Friday, I weighed 147.8 pounds. I reached my goal, however, my next Friday's goal would be 146.8 pounds; the goal weight reached less one pound—not the lower weight during the week.

These are the different scenarios for when and how to reach your weekly goals!! Hopefully, you noticed that I tried to come up with every possible way to reach the weekly goal! But, let's say that for some reason you do not meet your weight loss goal for the week—do not beat yourself up—things happen. Go through your journals and look at what you ate, when you ate, how much you slept, and then check your exercise journal to see if you included both aerobics and weight bearing exercises and did some physical activity every day. My guess is that you will find some areas in which were not your best efforts. Just resolve to do your best next week, and keep your next week's goal based on the following scenario.

If your goal was to be 165.4 pounds, and on Friday and during the week, you never got below 166.2 pounds, then your next Friday goal would be 165.2 pounds—one pound less the lowest amount reached during the week. If you have more than a couple of these types of weeks, look over your list of what your original motivation was, and make sure these motivators are still applicable. You may need to rewrite your motivators, or maybe just seeing the list of reasons for starting this journey may help you get going again. Either way, make sure you are still committed to your goals. *Chapter 6—Pitfalls During the Process*, will go over in more detail how to handle setbacks.

You may wonder what your reward is for reaching your weekly

goal. *You did it! Congratulations! You're the best! Awesome! Great job!* Write whatever comes to mind in your journal next to your achieved goal. Do not reward yourself with food, things, relaxation, partying, or anything else you may be tempted to give yourself. Feel the satisfaction of losing weight without feeling the need to get something for doing it. There are several reasons for this. One is that you may decide that what you would give to yourself this week is not really worth giving up that second helping of your mom's amazing lasagna. This is not good and becomes anti-motivating. Perhaps, you may not have a lot of money, so the fact that you cannot reward yourself the way that you feel you should or your friend rewards herself makes you sad. Don't be sad; you made your goal! Be happy!

Another reason not to reward yourself for losing weight is that you may need to have the thing you said would be your reward—but if you don't make your goal, what do you do? You really need a dress for the office party, and nothing fits, but you didn't make your goal for the week. Do you decide not to go to the party, because you can't buy a dress that fits, or do you buy a dress anyway and teach yourself that you will give yourself the reward even if you don't reach your goal? See there is no good solution. This does not mean that I don't want you to do nice things for yourself—I really do—but not because you reached a weight loss goal. Do things for yourself as often as you can. Create a list of things that you want or like to do, be sure to include items that do not cost anything and items that can be done at a moments notice. Maybe you like massages, giving yourself a pedicure, buying yourself a dozen roses, taking a walk along the beach, or buying a dress for a particular party—whatever it is, do them as often as you want. But do them because they are for you, and you deserve to do things that make you happy!

So are you ready for—*How to Do It?* I hope so, it's my favorite chapter!

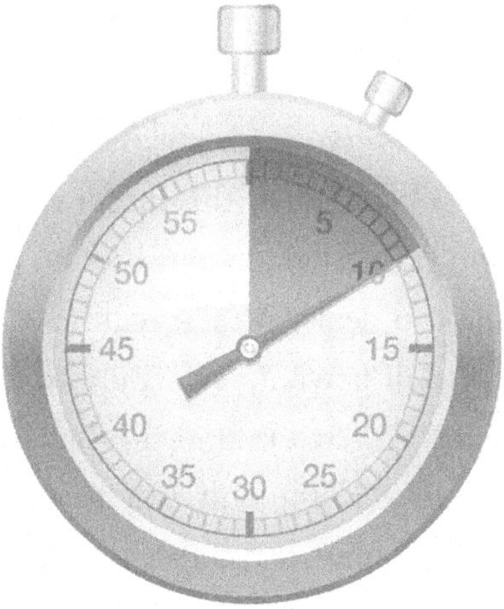

Chapter 5

How to Do It!

I had preconceived ideas about this chapter when I first began writing this book; I need to start by sharing some information about me that recently occurred that I thought would never happen. I had to make the decision to file for bankruptcy; I guess the decision was made for me when my largest client went out of business leaving me with a six-figure receivable and no other options to pay all of the bills. So here I am writing to you about how to lose weight, and while I have managed to keep my weight steady during this whole ordeal, having money to put groceries in the refrigerator is more on my mind than anything else. All my credit cards have been shut down, and I have very little money to my name. I used all of my savings, retirement funds, and investments to support myself while hoping that my biggest client would persevere and be as prosperous as he once was back in the day when home prices went up every week and there were lotteries just to see if you were allowed to bid on a home. *(As you can imagine there are tears running down my cheeks as I am writing this.)*

I bring all of this up for many reasons: (1) Life is unpredictable—you can set out on a mission to do things a certain way; yet you always have to deal with the realities that life gives to you. Don't be hard on yourself if what you set out to do isn't working; just adapt, figure out what will work, and do that instead, (2) I used to believe expensive foods were the only way to eat healthy—now I know that is not the case; I have learned a lot about healthy food options while on an extremely tight budget that I would not have otherwise, and (3) To let you know where my heart and thoughts are right now—*(a) how did I get here?, (b) what could I have done differently?, and (c) once I go through this bankruptcy what will I do different? So I never find myself here again!* The last item is something that we all have to look at when we are dealing with situations that have gotten away from us and we are now taking steps to get under control.

> *How did I get here? How do I make sure it doesn't happen again? What do I need to do to not gain the weight back? This introspection is essential and will give you the steadfastness needed to persevere in your journey.*

Let's get started on your journey of losing weight. You really must think of it as a journey. No two days will be the same, no one thing to eat is the trick, and no specific exercise will get you there. Stay the course, deal with detours along the way, and you *will* reach your destination—*assuming, of course, you know where you are going.* That is it for metaphors for now!

You Are Ready!

You have selected your method for tracking your nutrition and exercise. It has a place to record what and when you ate, how much you weigh every day, and the exercises you have done. You know how much weight you want to lose, and you can visualize what size clothes you will be in. You have set a realistic goal of how long it will take to get you there. You have plenty of clothes in the size you are currently wearing that you feel comfortable in and look good on you. You haven't told anyone that you are planning on losing weight!

> *No one should really notice you are trying to lose weight, since you are eating normal foods—just smaller amounts and more often. If someone notices that you didn't eat as much as you normally do, just say, "You know, I ate a few hours ago, and I guess I am just not as hungry as I thought." That is all true; there is no need to announce anything!*

Where Are You Starting From?

This is the moment of truth. How much do you weigh? Establish your *never again* number—five pounds more than what you weigh now. These numbers will continue to decrease as you lose weight, but they will never go up! Your *YIKES!* number is four pounds more than you are now, and your *OMG* number is three pounds more than you are now. Record *OMG!* or *YIKES!* in your journal next to your weight, if you reach either of them during the week.

Only weigh yourself in the morning upon voiding your bladder. If more than 15 minutes has gone by or you drank something before you remembered to get on the scale, do not weigh yourself that morning. Once you are into the habit of weighing yourself, it will get easier.

It is important to have a scale that gives you consistent results. If you get on and off the scale three times and get different numbers, you are not getting an accurate reading. This could be because of your scale, or it could be the place where the scale sits. Find a place that works for you. If it is your bathroom—great! If not, be sure your scale is somewhere you will remember to weigh yourself every morning before you start your day. Remember, it is not about how much you weigh today; it is about knowing where you are and tracking your progress to where you are going!

Write It Down

Enter your weight in your journal before you get too far into your day. I keep mine in my kitchen in a leather binder that matches the décor. If I have company, I can close it and either put it away with the cookbooks or leave it on the counter as if it were my appointment book.

You will want to go back to this information throughout your journey. Sometimes you will be amazed by how far you have come. Maybe you started out exercising 15 minutes a day, which was difficult at first, but now you easily log 60 minutes a day and wonder what the fuss was all about. Maybe you see how getting more sleep helped you lose weight—or that after nights when your sleep schedule was a little skimpy, the weight just didn't seem to budge.

Look over your journal often so you can see what worked and what did not. What made you feel good at the end of each meal? What made you feel tired or just not at your best? It is only once you start to write down your daily eating and exercise activities that you will get to know yourself!

I cannot stress this enough: everyone is different. Some people will feel better eating certain foods, and other people will feel better eating something completely different. The same goes with exercise—some people swear by running, but I personally cannot stand it—it hurts my body *all over.* However, I love a brisk walk on or off the treadmill; I feel very relaxed afterward.

Why do I care and what is important to write down?

» To make sure that each week includes a variety of different foods

» To make sure the foods have the intended effect—to either lose or maintain weight, feel calm and not dizzy

» To look back at eating intervals—waiting too long to eat can derail any weight loss plan. Sometimes it takes looking over the last week or two to see a pattern.

» You will have a higher success rate of writing it down if you write down what you ate before you eat it—while you are hungry, motivated, and might have extra time waiting for your food to be ready. Once you are done eating there is little motivation to record what you ate. (The start time is what your timer will be based on for your next meal)

What I do not care about and why you should not write it down!

» *Do not write down how much you ate.* Just because today you ate half a cup of cottage cheese and a quarter-cup of strawberries for a meal or mini-meal doesn't mean that tomorrow or next week, you should eat the same food in the same amount. Remember, every meal and every day is different, and your body will tell you how much to eat. Besides, you may not have eaten all of it. Saying "less three bites of this and two bites of that" is really not useful information.

» *Do not write down how many calories you ate*—again, it doesn't matter; you are only eating until you are satisfied, not until you reached a certain caloric intake. Also, assuming you believed in calories in/calories out, it is time consuming and practically impossible to obtain completely accurate information on how many calories you are taking in and burning every day—so why try?

» *Do not write down how many grams of dietary fat, protein, or carbohydrates you consumed.* It is not because it doesn't matter as much as it is really impossible to know for sure—then it just becomes useless information that you spent a lot of time trying to figure out. Keep it simple.
» *Do not write down a new entry if you finished eating less than 20 minutes ago and decided you were still hungry.* Say it is 12:15 pm, and you have made a simple lunch of cottage cheese and pineapple that takes you 10 minutes to eat. You think you have finished, but within 15 minutes, you think, *I wish I had some crunch with my meal; I just don't feel satisfied yet.* So you eat a couple of crackers with some goat cheese—just add those entries to your 12:15 pm meal.

Although I do not write down my feelings all the time—mostly when I am not feeling well or when I feel absolutely amazing after eating something—there is a lot to learn from doing so. When you write down how you feel after you have eaten, you will have a better insight into how certain combinations of foods or certain meals affect you. When I first started in my journey, I wrote down a lot of notes, such as "I ate too much", "still hungry", "decided to eat more", "felt dizzy, so I ate", and "felt stressed, so I ate".

I think now is a good time to state the obvious: there are a lot of reasons to eat! Being dizzy, cranky, stressed, or even boredom may be valid reasons to eat. It just depends on what you eat and how much you eat. But, if you are eating and it is not because you are hungry—write down why you *think* you are eating!

Measurements in Your Journal

When I started out on my journey I thought it would be interesting to know what my measurements were and how I was progressing. I was very curious about my midsection, so that is what I started measuring and what I use when I am on business trips to keep my weight in check. From there I moved on to measuring my right arm, right upper thigh, rib cage, hips, and waist once in a while. I don't do it often, and I don't recommend doing it more than once a month. You will want the difference to be measurable, and if it has only changed a sixteenth of an inch in the last couple of days, you aren't going to be that excited. Save measuring yourself for times when you have dropped a dress size or when you go on business trips, or keep it to once a month—or just don't do it!

Create Your Own Rules

So what should you *not* eat? First, figure out what your trigger foods are. Trigger foods are those foods that for some unexplained reason, you cannot eat a set amount that *you* decided on. Pringles and Goldfish crackers are my trigger foods. I don't buy them unless I am at a hotel and they are in the minibar. They are the little packages that are very expensive, but I know I am making a choice, and I sometimes decide I want to go ahead and indulge. I keep it to a confined time and place—on vacation or a business trip, in small amounts, and so expensive I do not want to eat more of them.

Most everyone has a trigger food. Maybe it's Junior Mints at the theater or a Snickers bar that calls you from the vending machine. You need to establish your own rules that you want to live by. If you go to the theater every weekend, eating Junior Mints every weekend is not such a great idea. Instead, make it a little harder by picking a number like three and on every weekend that has a three in the date, you can eat some Junior Mints.

If you're tempted by the vending machine, bring in cheese and fruit to work, but allow yourself to eat from the vending machine if (and only if) you just were too busy to get to the store and weren't able to bring your cheese and fruit to the office. Life is really unpredictable, and you can't and shouldn't say "never" to your trigger foods—it gives them too much power. Just try to make a game out of it and remember you do not need to eat all of it!

I go to a lot of conferences that have a fully catered lunch or dinner which always includes dessert that is sitting at the table when I first arrive. When I was on my journey losing weight, I set up a rule that said if the dessert was chocolate then I could eat some. Anything else, I would just leave it and not even consider eating it. I let fate be the decider for me. If there was chocolate on the table I knew I was having dessert and I ate accordingly and conversely if there wasn't I knew that I was not. I didn't feel any anguish over the decision because it was already decided a long time ago. The same for bread, if it was warm sourdough bread with butter; I would eat some, anything else I would not—no worries when the bread plate came around, my rules were already established.

Have a mantra to say to yourself when you are struggling with a decision. My mantra is, "*Not in my best interest*"—I like this one, because I still have the ability to choose. I know it is not the best choice for me and there is a better choice. Find a mantra that works for you!

How Often and How Much to Eat

This is where a timer is going to be your best friend. You want to eat anywhere from 2–4 hours apart. This seems like a big variation, but every day is different, every mealtime is different, and every person is different. If you are not used to eating at least four to five times a day, you will need to set your timer. I recommend setting your timer anyway just so you remind yourself that it is time to eat and your subconscious doesn't have to keep thinking about it. Have you ever had an upcoming meeting that was hours away or a project that was due but you weren't ready to start it and yet you kept thinking about it in your head over and over so you wouldn't forget about it? Well, the best way to forget and not worry about it anymore is to record it in your calendar with a reminder notification; your mind will keep thinking about something that it doesn't want *you* to forget. If you are constantly thinking about whether it is time to eat yet or forgetting to eat—set your timer.

If you are worried you will be hungry sooner vs. later, then set your timer for 2–2½ hours from the last time you *started* eating, not when you last finished your meal. Since we are only writing down when we start, we do not care when we stop; therefore, your timer will always be based on when your last meal started. If you are used to only eating once or twice a day (some people eat like this), then you are going to want to set your timer to 3½–4 hours from the last time you ate. This should let you feel like some time has passed, and you can go about your business not concerning yourself as to when you will need to eat your next meal.

> *Some people may think there is a lot of eating going on here and if they just cut out some of the intervals, they will lose even more weight—this is not true. Your body needs to have food on a consistent basis. This will affect your metabolism,*

> *ability to think, moods, and ability to cope with stress. Most importantly, frequent eating will help prevent you from overeating; which is really what causes weight gain.*
>
> *When you overeat, you are stretching your stomach. This in turn means that the next time you go to eat; there is more room and thus a need for more food in order for you to feel full. It becomes a continuing problem unless you are able to shrink your stomach. The healthiest way to shrink your stomach is to eat smaller portions throughout the day at shorter intervals.*

What if it has been less than two hours since your last meal and you are already hungry? Don't worry! First, be sure you aren't thirsty. If you have been drinking water throughout the day, this shouldn't be the issue, but if you haven't been sipping on water, try drinking about two ounces of cold water. If after 10 minutes, you are still hungry, then go ahead and eat something small that is primarily protein and dietary fat and has minimal carbohydrates (like an ounce of cheese). You may need to reset your timer again. Write down what you ate, and make a note that you were really hungry! Check to see what you ate last and make sure it was not too high in carbohydrates. If it was, then make a note of that particular dish and plan to add a little more protein and/or dietary fat as needed next time to even it out.

These journals are for your education, not to make you feel bad or accountable. I hate that word—*accountable.* I am an adult, I make my decisions, and I don't need to be accountable for what I eat! If you are hungry, you are hungry; you don't need to explain it, but you do want to write in your journal what your thoughts are as to why you feel hungry when *you* don't think you should be. If you think you are writing everything down to be accountable, you may lie to yourself! That is just counterproductive.

This is a journey—your journey. You need to learn about yourself and how your body reacts to eating certain combinations of foods and how your exercise helps your efforts. Maybe you are under a lot of stress for a certain project. This can make you hungry, and your brain is counting on you to feed it so it can keep going. Or, is it possible you are bored? Write something down beside the meal to help you decide if you are eating enough each time you eat and if you ate the right pro-rata of dietary fat, protein, and carbohydrates. Texture is important—maybe you just need some crunch—especially if boredom is your reason for wanting to eat.

How to Not Overeat

You may not realize that you have been overeating; unless you make a concerted effort to listen to your body it is easy to do. Some people eat too fast and there is not enough time for the feeling of satisfied to be triggered. I do not believe in the philosophy that you need to eat very slowly and chew your food a certain amount of times. Meals should be enjoyed in a relaxed environment and not require a lot of thought. However, if you find you are constantly eating so fast that you don't remember eating and it is affecting your waist line—then slow it down a *little*. Savor each bite just a little bit longer and enjoy your meal. If you are with others, take a moment to rest and talk with the other person in a casual manner.

At first it will take some trial and error, to understand when your body has had enough. This is my trick! If I had to eat again in an hour and half—could I? I started this by thinking what if my boyfriend calls, and asks if I want to grab a bite to eat? Normally he would be at least an hour from being ready to go. Then we would need to be seated and then order and our food delivered—so about an hour and a half. The way this started is that I didn't want him to know I was losing weight and I didn't want to say that I just ate and could not go out to eat.

The feeling you are going for when you finish eating is nothingness. This may sound really odd if you are reading this for the first time. But, it is the best way I can describe when you have a satisfying meal.

» You don't feel full or stuffed
» You don't feel like you are on a sugar high
» You don't feel heavy from too much dietary fat
» You don't feel anything—just comfortable

This next part may seem contradictory to what I have said before—that you should not let someone else tell you when to eat—but if four hours have gone by and you just don't feel hungry, aren't sleeping (don't wake yourself up to eat), aren't already scheduled to eat soon—then go ahead and eat something. How much you eat will depend on your appetite and what other eating commitments you have scheduled. Perhaps a mini-meal that is well-balanced—maybe a quarter of an apple with some peanut butter or a handful of mixed nuts (not all nuts are well-balanced so read the label). If you continually wait more than four hours between meals, you will impede your weight loss, plain and simple. If this seems to happen often, make sure you are not getting too much dietary fat at your meals. Look over your journal and see if that is possible. If it is, then add a little more protein and carbohydrates for a more balanced meal next time you eat.

Planning your day the way you would like it to be is the best way to start out. After a while, it will become a lot easier to fit in all the meals you need to eat. Again, every day holds a different set of circumstances. Work within those circumstances, and make a plan that works for you. Here are *examples* of lifestyles you may encounter and how to make a plan with an *example* menu for each—as always do not eat more than you are comfortable with—eat until just satisfied, *not* full.

Office Work—Monday through Friday

I normally have a *Sporadic Lifestyle*; however I spent an entire summer while writing this book working in an office for 10–12 hours a day from Monday–Thursday and a little less on Fridays. I felt very fortunate to have this experience when I did, because it reminded me of the different needs that people working in an office environment have. The main thing I learned quickly was the need to avoid the office foods like donuts, bagels, or homemade goodies that were brought in by well-intentioned people. Whenever you are offered these derailing foods, you can say, "Thank you so much, but I just ate." The best part is that it will probably be true!

- » **Breakfast:** Depending on your style and time available (most breakfasts take less than five minutes to make), you can do either of the following:
    - › Make breakfast and eat at home (example breakfast)
        - Canadian bacon
        - Egg with butter
        - Toast with butter (melted before you put it on the toast)
            - » It is important to melt the butter so you put less on. It will satisfy you more, since it will be warm and get into the bread.
        - Slice of an orange (this is like a garnish—approximately a quarter-inch thick)
    - › Make breakfast and eat on the go
        - Toast very lightly with butter (so it can bend easily)
        - Egg and cheese omelet

  - Put the omelet on the toast and wrap it in aluminum foil
  - Wrap in paper towels so you don't drip on yourself
- › Buy breakfast on your way to work—something with egg, ham, cheese, and bread. I ate the breakfast *ham, cheddar cheese and parmesan frittata on an artisan roll* at Starbucks many a morning along with a *peppermint mocha* (I was in maintenance mode at the time and I only ate and drank until the point of being satisfied, not full)

» **Midmorning mini-meal:** This should take less than 10 minutes to make, eat, and clean up.

- › Bring enough food for the entire week and keep it in the refrigerator
  - Hard-boiled eggs
  - Deli meat, thinly sliced
  - Cheese slices
  - Grapes or cherries
- › Buy something from the cafeteria or coffee shop at your office
  - Cottage cheese with pineapple
  - Hard-boiled egg
- › If you don't have a refrigerator or coffee shop available, bring nonperishable foods and keep them in your drawer.
  - Mixed nuts
  - Almonds (there are a lot of seasoned almonds to choose from)
  - Beef jerky

- **Lunch:**
    - Bring your own lunch
        - Leftovers from the previous night's dinner
        - Sandwich with or without bread and a little fruit
            - The breadless sandwich is deli meat, cheese slice; rolled up (with or without condiments)
    - Go out for a sit-down lunch
        - Know the best options from the menus of restaurants you frequent—save your favorite selections somewhere easily accessible (like your phone), so you can select from your own predetermined choices instead of the menu when you are at the restaurant.
    - Fast food
        - Every fast food restaurant has options that will work with your plan. Some options may require a little adjustment, like not eating sauces. (Sauces usually have a lot of sugar in them.) Maybe just eat half of what you normally would get.

- **Late afternoon mini-meal:** Since you ate a well-balanced meal during lunch, you should not be dragging during the afternoon. But you still need to eat again sometime midafternoon. The same options available for the midmorning mini-meal will work for the late afternoon mini-meal as well. Here are some additional ideas:
    - Broccoli and cheese sticks
    - Celery and peanut butter
    - Prosciutto and cantaloupe

- **Additional mini-meal:** Some people like to eat late; other people like to eat early, I can tell you that it doesn't matter when it comes to weight loss. I routinely eat after 7:00 pm, and I have been known to eat as late as 9:00 pm and as early as 5:00 pm. If you know you are going to eat very late, just add another mini-meal into your early evening so that you do not let more than 3–4 hours pass between meals. If you have dinner early in the evening you may need to add a mini-meal in between when you go to bed and dinner.

We will talk more about dinner and late evening later on, since it is the same for everyone, regardless of lifestyle. Dinner ideas are included in *Appendix C—Menus and Restaurant Guide*

Sporadic Lifestyle

Some lifestyles are more open and every day is different. I truly understand that lifestyle and can share what I have learned.

- **Breakfast:** Eat breakfast within 1½ hours of waking—time can come and go quickly if you aren't careful. Set your timer, and make sure you eat breakfast within the first 1½ hours upon waking.

  I love to drink my coffee before I eat, but I used to find myself on a call with a client or need to deal with some issue that came through via e-mail, and the next thing I knew, it had been more than two hours since I had woken up and I still hadn't eaten.

- **Midmorning mini-meal:** Depending on what time I wake up, this might be skipped, since I sometimes wake up around 9:00

am. If I eat breakfast by 10:30 am, I am usually ready for lunch around 1:00 pm or so. A midmorning snack is only needed if you wake up early in the morning and there would be more than 3–4 hours between eating breakfast and lunch.

» **Lunch:** Sometimes I have client meetings or conference lunches so I am at the whim of the choices I am given—I try to stick with meat, chicken, fish and a salad (rarely will I drink alcohol at a business lunch—it is no longer anticipated that business people will drink at lunch, so avoid doing so, if possible).

If I am at my home office, I go to my menus—normally I just want to make something quickly and get back to work. Here are some quick and easy lunches that allow me to keep working:

› Leftovers are easy and quick
› Sandwich with a small piece of fruit (I toast my bread for crunch)
› Salads with precooked chicken strips

» **Late afternoon mini-meal:** This is a must for me, since I eat dinner late. I really need to make sure that I eat something in the late afternoon.

› Watermelon and blue cheese
› Goat cheese spread *thickly* on crackers
› Almonds and fresh cherries
› Cottage cheese and pineapple

» **On the go:** (anytime of the day)

› Cheese Stick (can be in your purse)
› Chicken pieces *without sauce*—fast food
› Individual pack of almonds

Active, On Your Feet Lifestyle

If you spend your day on your feet—possibly due to your job—you will have different challenges. Since I was a cashier at a grocery store many moons ago, I remember some of the issues that can arise.

- **Breakfast:** Before you head out, be sure to eat a hearty breakfast! This is extremely important, since you are probably only going to be able to eat during your break and at lunch.
  - Eat at home—eggs, Canadian bacon, toast with butter, and a small amount of fruit, such as two strawberries
  - Eat on the run—something with eggs, cheese, ham, and bread

- **Midmorning and late afternoon mini-meals:** You may not have access to a refrigerator, so you want to think of foods you can keep with you.
  - Beef jerky
  - Almonds
  - Mixed Nuts
  - Cashews

- **Lunch:**
  - If you are able to bring your lunch and have a refrigerator then follow the *Office Work Lifestyle*
  - If you need to buy your lunch every day then it will be important for you to go to the websites of the various restaurants you have to choose from and pick out several options that will work for you
  - If you bring your lunch but do not have access to a

refrigerator, then you will need to be creative. Here are some ideas:

- Peanut butter with a banana or an apple
- Tuna kits that you make at lunch
- Nuts and beef jerky

If you are able to bring a small cooler with you your choices will open up immensely. Be sure to have a refrigerator thermometer in your cooler, so you know the temperature is appropriate for what you are keeping.

Dinner Dates and Events

If you have dinner plans or an evening event to go to, then you can back into your daily eating schedule by figuring out when you will eat dinner. Keep in mind that even if you are to meet someone for dinner at 7:00 pm, that does not mean you will eat at 7:00 pm, so factor in that you are going to need to wait for the other person, wait for the table, wait to have your order taken and your food served.

My boyfriend is *always* 15 minutes late. I know this and plan for it. Then I factor in that we will probably have a cocktail before dinner, so I try to eat half an ounce of cheddar cheese about 1–1½ hours before our meeting time. In this case, we are going to meet for dinner at 7:00 pm; I figure he will get there at 7:15 pm and that we will have a drink. We will probably have a salad or appetizer around 7:45 pm, so I will have half an ounce of cheese around 6:00 pm so I am not on edge and won't be starving when it comes time to eat. At dinner I only eat what I really feel comfortable eating. I usually have leftovers. If I want to have dessert, then I make sure I leave a little room. I feel like I have compartments—one for salad, one for the entrée, and then of course, one for dessert. (I don't always have dessert—if I feel like it, I do and if I don't, then I don't—regardless, I would not eat an entire dessert by myself, and I do not take dessert home as leftovers.)

Right before Bedtime

Depending on what time you eat dinner and go to bed, you may need to have cheese and saltine crackers right before you go to bed. If I go to bed within two hours of having dinner, I don't need to eat something right before bed. Normally, I eat anywhere from one to four saltine crackers with cheddar cheese (cut about an eighth-inch thick) on them. If you make too many, just don't eat them!

You do not want to go to bed hungry. One of the worst feelings I remember from being on other diets is going to bed hungry. I just won't do it anymore. It was one of the things that I originally wrote down that I did not like about other diets that I used to reverse-engineer this program. I wasn't sure at first what would happen, but I also knew I did not want to go to bed hungry, since it would keep me from sleeping. Then I wouldn't get enough sleep, and that would keep me from losing weight.

With faith in what I knew to be true for me, I began my weight loss journey eating cheddar cheese and saltine crackers before I went to bed, and I lost all the weight I wanted to and more. I have never deviated from allowing myself to eat before bed. Sometimes I have dinner so late that I don't feel the need to eat cheese and crackers before I go to sleep, but I never go to bed hungry! You shouldn't go to bed hungry either!

Water

Make sure you drink enough water—take it with you wherever you go! What constitutes "enough" is based on your personal situation—do not drink so much that you feel full, thus stretching your stomach.

If your urine is a dark yellow, you must drink more water until it is a light yellow on a continual basis. While eight 8-ounce glasses of water is the expected norm, you really need to take into account all the other liquids you drink, your activity level, and various other factors like weather—just keep hydrated. I hope you decided to give up drinking soda and other sugary drinks on a daily basis, which would leave you with coffee, tea, and water—and yes alcohol is allowed on the *Timer* DIET program.

There are a lot of different kinds and brands of water. There is bottled water that comes in plastic or glass, flat vs. sparkling, filtered water, well water, soft water, tap water, and reverse osmosis water. I wish I knew the answer as to which kind was better or worse for you, but I don't. I can't use the charcoal filter that is in some filtered water; it affects my throat adversely. I don't think that sparkling (bubbly) water is best to drink as your daily water, but for special dinners, it is fine.

There have been a lot of studies about plastic water bottles getting hot and adversely affecting the water, so I am sure to never leave my water in the car! I pick my bottle up and put it in my purse no matter how long I will be gone. (I live in Phoenix, so the car can heat up 40 degrees in just minutes during the summer.) I have started being more eco-conscious and drinking cold water (no ice—it can affect the taste) from a large glass or plastic bottle at home. I drink it out of a nice glass; for some reason it tastes better than out of an individual bottle.

You can get testing kits to see if your tap water is good to drink. As important as it is to drink water, I wish that there was a foolproof way to know that the water you drink is good for you. I don't think it is possible to be completely sure. Do not let this deter you from drinking water. Adding flavors to your water is not needed—if your water does not taste good, look into a different water supply. If you live in a dry climate, like I do, you may need to drink water during the night as well.

Desserts

If you are in the habit of having dessert with every single meal, reassess this, and see if this is the best thing for you right now in your weight loss journey. Is it something you will want to go back to after you lose the weight you want? Here is my feeling on the topic; if you feel that dessert at dinner is a part of your life (maybe a ritual—that is not adversely affecting anyone else) and you know you will go back to eating dessert every night once you lose the weight, then I say you need to keep it in your current weight loss plan. (You weren't expecting that—were you?)

Having a small dessert after dinner or lunch will not derail your weight loss efforts: If you stop eating desserts while you are losing weight and then as soon as you are ready to maintain you can't wait to go back to eating them at every meal, you will gain back the weight pretty quickly. The other possibility is that you will feel deprived during your weight loss journey and either give up or feel like you gave in when you have dessert. Guilt is not good when you are on your weight loss journey.

If you decide to incorporate dessert make it small, fresh, and delicious. No fat-free, sugar-free, or "good for you" dessert! Most importantly, enjoy each bite, slowly taking in the taste and the smell. Make it memorable and guilt-free! Have your dessert within 30 minutes of eating your last bite of dinner. The protein from your dinner is needed to offset your dessert, so don't wait too long. You can always decide to have dessert tomorrow—which sometimes is the best decision.

Eating Foods You Like

It is very important to like the foods you eat. Experimenting can be exciting or intimidating. I like trying new types of fish when I eat out, since trying to make fish at home—especially for the first time—can be intimidating. If your relationships are such that asking for a bite of someone else's meal is acceptable, go for it! What better way to try out a new food than committing to just one taste?

If you try a food and don't like it, just don't eat anymore. I recommend trying new foods whenever the option is made available. Also, revisit some of those foods you remember not liking as a child. When I was growing up, my stepfather made salmon patties, and they were disgusting. One time, I got food poisoning from them and couldn't even imagine eating salmon again in my life! But in my late twenties, I was at dinner and someone asked if I wanted to try some fresh grilled salmon. I went ahead and agreed to have a taste. I was amazed, it was awesome! I still stay away from salmon patties, but decided other types of salmon were actually worth trying. Now I love many types of salmon: smoked, grilled, baked, seasoned, and unseasoned. I would have missed out on an amazing fish if I never allowed myself to get past my childhood memories.

If you have kids at home, you are helping them make memories, too. Make your journey fun and enjoyable, and they will learn by example. Eating great foods that are also good for you can be the best nutritional education you can give to your children.

Presentation

Sometimes you have the time for presentation and a pretty plate that looks amazing with garnishes and such, and at other times, you don't. If you made the choice to buy new dishes, you should have dishes that are the right size for the situation. If not, you still want a variety of sizes. Buying a few smaller plates and bowls may be a good idea. There are certain things you want to do and do not want to do when it comes to presentation. You don't want a large 12-Inch plate when you are eating half a sandwich. If at all possible you want no more than an inch or two of the side of the plate showing. Use small bread plates for your crackers and cheese or other mini-meals. You can also use your custard cups for a mini-meal of cottage cheese and fruit. You want your dish to fit your meal—not too big and not too small!

Do not eat or drink out of a container—not a cottage cheese container, ice cream container, or milk or juice out of the carton. Why is this so important? When you do this, you treat your body like a trash can! You empty out a food or drink into your body. You are not giving your body the respect that it deserves by putting the food or drink into a bowl, in a glass, or on a plate. You deserve better than to treat yourself like a trash can, so don't do it!

Exercise

Why do you want to exercise? You may say you don't really *want* to. Is that true? The benefits of exercise appear to be significant—better memory, warding off various diseases, relief of stress, a better night's sleep, better sex drive, increased muscle tone, increased metabolism, and perhaps most importantly—aging better. Which of these benefits do not appeal to you?

What would you rather do for thirty minutes to an hour every day instead of exercise that produces the same benefits? Some of us would rather watch TV—*workout in front of the TV.* Some of us would rather play with our kids—*play in an active way with your children.* Even infants can be taken for a walk in a stroller and after a few months they can be part of a "mom and me" yoga or strength training program. Some of us say we are just always running around—*do your walking with some vigor.* When you are out shopping, carry your bags and switch arms, especially if you are carrying children. My favorite thing is to do something with my doggie, Princie—we play tug-of-war or play ball, go for walks or pulls (as he likes to do)! Don't worry if you don't have the money to get a gym membership or a four legged friend to get you moving—you have a home and a body, you have a home gym!

I found in the past I have succumbed to the delusion that I could buy an exercise video or piece of equipment and think, *I am going to get into shape!* I forgot that buying something did not *get* me into shape. Try as I might to make the osmosis thing work for me, it did not! So yes, you do have to put forth effort, but fortunately, momentum is on your side. Once you start excising, you will actually start to crave it. This is one of the reasons that I say you need to workout every day. You want it to be something that you really miss if you miss a day. If you start working out aerobically you will find the stress relief is so great that the next time you are having a stressful time, you will want to take a break and do something to exert yourself so you feel better and clear your head. Brisk walking is a great way to start out exercising!

I have a few cautions before starting to exercise. You would think safety is surely a concern and it is. But I would like to start with the most insidious way that exercise may play havoc with your weight loss journey: *You may think you burned more calories than you really did.* I truly recommend that you don't even pay attention to how many calories your machine says you are burning or some magazine says that running for 30 minutes burns. It doesn't really matter. In fact not only does it not matter how many calories you burned, more than likely how many calories you *think* you burned, you did not. This is not bad news. It is not good news either; it is just information that is useless and serves no real purpose in your journey.

When I used to look at the treadmill and realize that after a half hour, I had not even come close to burning 200 calories, I was disheartened. I even got to the point of wondering why I bothered to workout. Surely there were easier ways to reduce calories, like skipping dessert or a latte. *That's it—I'll skip my latte, and I won't need to exercise!* No! Regardless of anything else you have going on in your life, find time to exercise every day. It is good for you and it will improve your mood. Try to do something you really like at least once a week—maybe golf, racquetball with a friend, or soccer with the kids. You do not need to be on a treadmill inside with your headphones on, but you can if you want.

Take it slow at first. If you have not worked out routinely for the last 30 days, then start out with a 15 minute walk or some type of simple aerobic moves every day. Then you can introduce weights for five minutes a day. If you have to cut back your aerobics to 10 minutes because you can only find 15 minutes in each day to workout, then that is fine (for starters). Be sure to start out with weights slowly. Stretch the muscles you are going to work before you exercise, and then stretch again afterward. (See *Appendix D—Exercise* for examples) Maintain good form, and perform your movements so that they are slow and intentional. Do not go fast, allowing momentum to do the work for you; this can also lead to injury.

You should never workout on an empty stomach or in the morning before breakfast. The main reason is so that you do not find yourself in a situation where you are lightheaded and make either a mistake in your routine or trip and injure yourself. Whatever metabolic boost you may or may not get from working out before eating is not worth the risk of injuring yourself. It is also not worth the risk to do something you do not feel comfortable with. This includes taking the stairs when they seem a little deserted or parking as far away as possible when it is dark or just doesn't feel right. I know there are ways to get in a few more steps, but not all of them are safe—especially if you are out by yourself. Above all, be safe!

Workout every day! Why do I say every day instead of the traditional three times a week? There are some reasons: (1) your body was made to move every day, not just three times a week, (2) if you workout the same amount every day, your appetite will be more consistent, (3) when you only workout three times a week, it becomes very easy to keep putting it off—to the point that an entire week has gone by, and you didn't even workout once, and (4) if you do have to miss one day, you probably won't feel so guilty that you missed one day. Hopefully, you will miss working out!

There are many different ways to workout. Pick something that works with your schedule and personality and includes aerobics and resistance training. Mix it up! Also, have alternatives. If you want to play tennis and the person or persons you normally play with are not available for a certain scheduled session, be sure to have alternative workout plans so that you don't just skip it altogether. Maybe your thing is running outside. Be sure to have an indoor alternative for bad weather or maybe a season. I live in Phoenix, during the summer it is dangerous to be out during the day. I do a lot of indoor activities during the summer and during the cooler months; I go hiking, golfing, and rollerblading (always have water available when outside!).

> *Enjoy the seasons where you live! Snowboarding, gardening, water skiing, and picking up fall leaves are all excellent ways to exercise and celebrate the seasons.*

Ratio of Weight Resistance vs. Aerobics and Personal Trainers

If you have worked out aerobically routinely for at least two weeks, it is time to include weight resistance into your routine. The ratios for the time spent on weight resistance training would be one-third weight training and two-thirds aerobic activity. It's pretty simple. (If you only have time for one—then go for aerobic activity.)

A word of caution on personal trainers—they do not feel what you feel. If you feel you have gone too far, then you have gone too far.

Personal trainers may be good for motivation, but do not let them push you too far or too fast. You risk injury, which then results in setbacks, when someone else decides how far you should go. It is much better to go slow and steady toward your goals! Remember that your goals are what matters, not those of your personal trainer.

> *Back in the 90s I thought I would go to a personal trainer who insisted my goal must be to achieve 18 percent body fat. That just seemed crazy to me—I was very clear that was not my goal—again he insisted that if I wanted a personal trainer then I needed to aim for the best body possible (according to him all women should be at 18 percent body fat). I fired him on the spot!*

Do *not* buy into the "no pain, no gain" motto. If you are in pain, you are hurting your body; slow and steady will get you to your goals. Personal trainers are great if you have never worked out with free-weights before and do not know about proper form. They will also show you how to use all of the machines and can provide great ideas on workout routines. Just remember—*you* need to go slow and steady toward a fitter you!

How Often and How Long to Workout Each Day

Your particular circumstances will dictate how often and how long to workout each day. If you can plan for 30 minutes each day as your goal, that is good. If you can get up to 60 minutes each day, that is even better. Go gradually, and do not increase by more than 15 minutes daily—feel free to stay with a routine for a week or two before you increase your time again. Something else to keep in mind is that you do not need to workout all at once in a day. If you are only able to find 10 minutes three times a day to workout and you are really focused on your workout during those 10 minutes that is also good. If you can workout 20 minutes three times a day that is even better! Just remember to make time for your warm-ups and cool-downs. They don't take long, but they are important to do. (See *Appendix D—Exercise*)

Working Out Different Amounts of Time on Different Days

The ideal situation is to workout for the same amount of time every day, but not everyone is able to do this because of work or other commitments. Here is a little twist that may work into your schedule. I used this when I needed to work at the office for 8–12 hours a day Monday–Friday. For the days you have time commitments, workout 15 minutes each day (in my case Monday through Friday); on the weekend workout for 1½ hours each day (not necessarily all at once). It seemed to work; my weight stayed consistent and I felt good about the smaller amount of focused time I worked out during the week. I prefer to workout the same amount of time each day, but for the summer while I worked in the office, it seemed to be a great work-around.

Exercise Journal

Your exercise journal is the best place to create your routine. Change your routine every two to four weeks—more often in the beginning and less often as you become fit. Be sure to include aerobic activity and workout all of the muscles in your arms and legs by trading off each day for the two muscle groups. (Do weight-bearing exercises on your arms one day and legs the next—if you have, or are prone to varicose veins (heredity)—*do not do weight-bearing exercises on your legs*, instead focus on toning by using inclines on treadmills and walking up and down stairs.) Vary the type of exercise, amount of time (normally referred to as *reps*), and weight when you change your routine.

When doing three sets of weights (start by setting your timer for 30 seconds), start with your first set at your average ability. At first you will need to do some trial and error to see what weights you should be using. After you have established your weights it will be easier to increase them as you change your routines. For example: if at three pounds you can do one arm for 30 seconds easily, but at five pounds not as easily, however, certainly doable without strain, then do your first set at three pounds, your second set at five pounds (feel free to stop before the time is up if you need to), and if you feel a little tired, do only one pound for your third set, or do another set using three pounds if you feel you have enough energy. Always stop if you are feeling exhausted.

Below are some ideas for how to workout at home. Even if you prefer to workout at a gym or doing something outside, you want to be able to workout at home if the situation arises. Your best chance of success is to have as many obstacles already figured out so they do not derail you!

Appendix D—Exercise has detailed instructions, sample routines, and examples of how to move up in your routines as you progress.

Workout at Home without Equipment or Cost

» Dancing
» Twisting from side to side
» Jump rope (fake—you may break something inside using a real one)
» Push-ups
» Marching in place
» Walking around the house
» Tricep-dips (with a very sturdy chair on carpet—not a rug)

- Standing exercises
- Leg exercises

Workout at Home with Minimal Equipment and Cost

- Video workout
  - Step aerobics (step required)
  - Arm workout (weights needed)
- Weights of one, three, five, and eight pounds make a good starting set

> *Start with one-pound weights if you have not routinely worked with weights during the last 30 days. That may seem light, but you will increase your weights gradually—there is nothing gained by lifting more than you should and injuring yourself! Have the next weights up on hand so you are ready when it is time to increase your weights. I still love my one-pound weights. Even today, I add them to my workout on the recumbent bike!*

- Stretch/resistance bands
- Hula hoop
- Rollerblades—always wear all of the protective gear
- Yoga—you need some instruction whether a video, book, or person
- Jump rope outside

Workout at Home with Equipment

Sometimes turning one of the rooms in your home into a gym is the most cost effective and time efficient thing to do. I turned my family room into a home gym and loved it! (Admittedly, I had the home gym when I was gaining weight and just didn't use it very often—so just having a home gym will not cause you to lose weight—you must use it!) It was right next to the kitchen so if I was cooking I could be close by. There was a TV so I could catch up on my favorite entertainment shows while I worked out. If I wanted to sing while listening to the stereo or my iPod I could do so without bothering anyone. Before you invest in a gym membership consider creating a home gym complete with equipment. Check used sporting equipment stores for great deals (first look at the recall lists—to insure what you are considering does not pose a risk).

Items to consider in a home gym:

» Treadmill
» Stationary bike
» Elliptical machine (my personal favorite if you only have one machine)
» Bicycle
» Workout bench along with free weights (on a non-slip surface)

Workout Away From Home

If you are on vacation less than three weeks a year, you don't have to incorporate your written journal or exercise routine into your vacation. Just enjoy yourself, and include as many activities as possible (including walking), and remember, don't overeat! See *Chapter 8—Vacations and Business Travel* for more ideas to ensure you have a plan to stay on track while you are away.

Here are some workout ideas for while you are away from home:

» March in place. You don't have to stomp—just lift your legs up and down in the same place.

- » Walk around the hotel or inside the hotel. Always be aware of your surroundings, and take the advice of the hotel concierge or front desk regarding the hotel's safety.
- » Do tricep-dips on a very sturdy stationery chair only on carpet not on a rug, a sturdy bench at the foot of the bed—do not attempt these if you feel they cannot hold your weight! Also, do not attempt tricep-dips if you have not been working out your arms on a routine basis for at least a month. You do not want to risk injury and you must have *some* tricep muscles established before attempting them—start slowly!
- » Push-ups provide a great workout. Do as many as possible before you are at the point of physical fatigue. Do not allow yourself to collapse; you want to be in full control of your body with each push-up.
- » Crunches are **not** my favorite exercise when I am at home, but on the road, they are easy to do! If you are concerned about the floor, put down a bath towel. It is important to hold your abs in while you do crunches.
- » Stretch bands are the best thing to use while traveling for resistance training. They take up virtually no extra room in your suitcase, and you can carry one or more for a variety of workouts, including upper and lower body.

Working Out to Music, a Podcast, or TV

Sometimes I am a little slow when it comes to technology. The term "playlist" didn't occur to me until a few years after starting my weight loss journey. Now I love using my playlists to help me in my workout routine. I pick songs that I currently love. I have various playlists that last anywhere from 15 minutes to an hour to match how long I have to work out. Having a playlist will help you to not think about when your time is up, since you know that when the playlist is done, so is your exercise time. You can have a specific song be your last song in all of your playlists so you will always know you are getting close to the end of your workout! With or without a playlist, working out to music keeps you motivated, brightens the mood, and makes the time go faster!

I sometimes listen to a podcast when I work out and I want to do double duty, but if the content is something that I will need to stop and write, then it doesn't work very well. Consider what you are listening to while you work out—you don't want something stressful such as watching world crises while you are on the treadmill. Be in the moment and enjoy your workout. Sometimes it is best to just have fun and either listen to some music or watch some entertaining TV.

When to Workout

Some people swear by working out in the wee hours of the morning, and others don't even think about it until they have finished their day at work. There is no right time to workout. Whatever works for you is the best time. There is a wrong time to workout, and that is when you are too tired. If you are not a morning person and force yourself to start working out at 5:00 am before having your cup of coffee and a bite to eat, then you risk injury by doing something that goes against your nature. If you are the type of person who works so hard during the day that when you come home, you are exhausted, then exercising after a day at work is not the answer either.

Try to see when *your* personal energy level is at its best, and decide what works for you. You may be able to find time to take a 30 minute walk during your lunch hour and still have time to eat beforehand. This is great if it works for you! Remember it does not need to be done all at the same time.

If you feel like you are *always* tired, then try working out about half an hour after you get up in the morning. Have a small, well-balanced breakfast and cup of coffee (if that's your thing) first, and see if you can fit your exercise in then. Sometimes you just have to go forward and try working out!

Sleep

Sleep is so very important! I know this seems like a strong statement, but on days when I do not get a good night of solid sleep, I tend to gain weight, even now that I am maintaining. Be sure to get between seven and nine hours of sleep. If you are catching up due to traveling or having to work on a deadline and burned the midnight oil, then 10–11 hours is fine once in a while. The worst thing is to have interrupted sleep. It isn't a big deal if you need to get up and can go straight back to sleep; it does not seem to affect the sleep process. It is the times when you start thinking about life, finances, relationships, or work—when you need to be sleeping—that can cause problems in your weight loss journey.

What should you do? That depends whether this insomnia is chronic, temporary, or just sporadic. If it is sporadic—less than once or twice a month—then it may not be of any concern, sometimes there will be nights that are harder to get to sleep than others. If it is temporary—a few days in a row but not lasting more than a week—be sure you exercise daily but not when exhausted. If you are very tired, then walk briskly for your daily routine and skip the weights until you have your sleep schedule back to normal.

If your insomnia is chronic, seek help from your doctor or talk with someone who specializes in sleep disorders (going to a sleep clinic may be a possibility). There are many possible reasons for chronic insomnia—some physical and some psychological—so medical help is the best plan of action if this is your situation. Please do this as soon as you realize this is a chronic problem. Two weeks of ongoing insomnia would be considered cause for concern.

Some *ideas* to help you get optimal sleep:

» Stop having caffeine after 2:00 pm (This includes chocolate—if you are having sleep problems)
» Turn off electronic equipment at least one hour before you go to sleep—this includes phones, e-mail, computers, TVs, and all other electronic items—avoid items with a bright light for the hour prior to going to bed
» Read a book before going to sleep—a low level of light is best
» Write in a journal about events that are good and bad. Always write at least one thing you are grateful for, but don't hesitate to write down problems.
» Keep a pen and paper by your bedside so you can write down thoughts that go through your mind and keep you from sleeping.
» Don't forget to eat your cheese and crackers within half an hour or less of when you go to sleep; if you are hungry.
» Try out different aromatherapy sleep pillow mists or relaxation mists. Be sure to test them at the store to see if the scent really relaxes you. The relaxation effect should be instantaneous.
» Sleep on freshly washed or new sheets. You want to feel good in your bed, so if your sheets are pilling, then invest in some new ones. Washing your sheets once a week will make you feel more comfortable, too.
» Keep the bedroom cool, and add a blanket to snuggle under
» Consider a melatonin regimen—only after discussing with your doctor if you are able to do so and you are not currently

taking any other medications that would adversely interact with the melatonin (including, but not limited to birth control)

» Pray or meditate—an attitude of gratitude when you put your head on the pillow can create inner calmness

Another trick I learned over the years to feel more rested is to learn to wake up without an alarm. You can train yourself to do this by setting your alarm and tell yourself to wake up five minutes before your alarm is set to wake you. (So if your alarm is set to 6 am—say to yourself wake up at 5:55 am.) It may take a little time to learn; be consistent and stick with! It is fun to do!

Resting vs. Relaxation

Resting is different from sleep and different from relaxation—let me explain: Resting occurs when your eyes are closed, you are not moving, but you are not sleeping. Relaxation is anything that you enjoy doing. For some people, playing a musical instrument is relaxing—for others it is painting, writing, or golfing, etc. Resting is more passive, like a massage or facial, or sunbathing (once in a while). Incorporate resting and relaxation into your life. It's not always possible to do every day, but if you can incorporate them into your life and look forward to them, your life will be more enjoyable.

Checking Your Clothing Size

It is tempting to check to see if your smaller size jeans fit every day—but don't! Once you have lost about seven or eight pounds or your current jeans feel loose, take out all of your jeans in the lower size and the jeans you currently wear. Make a true assessment of fit, and make sure they are flattering. Loose jeans are not flattering, but neither are tight jeans.

You may keep some that you have been wearing and you may also bring in some of the smaller size jeans as well. The goal is to make sure you can go to your closet and feel confident that anything you pick fits you! Once you are done, pack away all the jeans you won't be wearing right now including the ones that are too big. Remember, they will be part of a cathartic activity later in *Chapter 9—Now that You Have Lost the Weight.*

If you need to buy clothes because you don't have enough of the size you currently are, just remember to not spend a lot of money on your purchases. Don't buy something so adorable that you will not be excited to get to a smaller size. Do not buy a lot of clothes! Even if you have the money to do so, don't do it—not yet!

Remember to check your bras and underwear after every 10–15 pounds of weight loss. They should be comfortable but not too loose or tight. When buying bras while losing weight, you can buy them so that they fit on the first hook, usually they will tell you to buy for the middle hook, but go ahead and get them if they fit well on the first hook— you will get more use out of them. If you need to buy new bras, don't buy a lot of them—just enough to get you through to the next time you need to change your bra size. These rules are not just for people who do not have a large clothing budget! You do not want to buy anything that will possibly hinder your progress—even subconsciously!

So these are the basics of *How to Do It!* What happens when there are bumps in the road, and you know there will be; at least I hope you are not expecting everything to go perfectly? Let's look at *Pitfalls During the Process …*

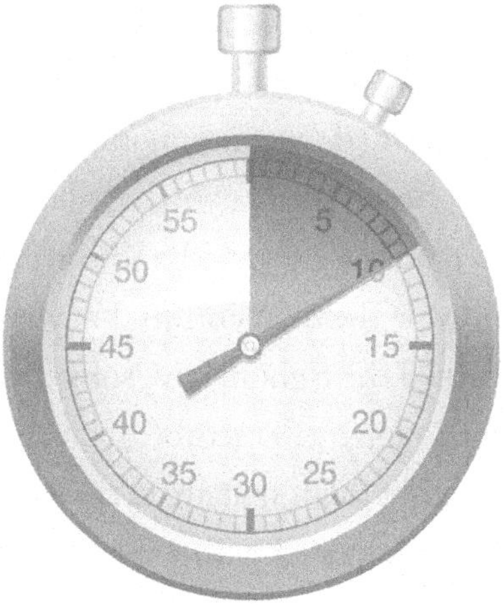

Chapter 6

Pitfalls During the Process

Breaking momentum is the biggest pitfall during the process that you will want to do what you can to either prevent or minimize, and if needed, get your momentum back. During any journey, there is momentum (the process of going forward), and there can be moments of stalling (going nowhere)—and worse, retraction (going backward). In the simplest of terms you are always doing one of the three.

You will usually find that in the beginning of any venture your ability to go forward is not so hard; in some cases, it can be effortless. As time goes on, it seems like it is not as easy and becomes discouraging. Perhaps you are *stalling*—going nowhere. If you don't take steps at this time in your journey, you may begin to retract and start to go backward. This may seem so simple and obvious that there is no reason to even mention it, but understanding the concept of momentum is the key to your ongoing success. (This is also why maintenance is so elusive—you are purposely stalling)

Why do we lose momentum? That, you must decipher as soon as it occurs! Is it that you have been losing weight so easily that you began to take it for granted and started eating foods that you know will not provide the momentum that you once enjoyed? Maybe you felt that you earned the right to have some indulgences, since you have been so good for so long. (Remember, you should always eat foods you enjoy while limiting foods that are *not in your best interest.*) Perhaps, something may have happened with your schedule, and you were not able to work out for an extended period of time. Or maybe you haven't been getting the sleep that you need to allow for the optimal recuperation time that is needed to keep your momentum.

The worst thing you can do at this stage is to say: *That's okay; it is to be expected; or there is nothing I can do about it!* There is a reason—I guarantee it! Get your journals out and look over them in detail. Go back to the time when you were losing weight and a few days before that. Then start checking your sleep, workout routine, times you ate, and what you ate. See if you find anything different that may have occurred. Is it possible that you stopped writing in your journal; and that in and of itself is what occurred? That is actually good news, because you can fix that right away!

Maybe the reason is more sinister. Did you eat more prepared foods or foods away from home that you know are *not in your best interest?* Maybe you waited too long to eat between meals, which then caused you to overeat once you had food in front of you. Maybe it was the season and there were too many parties in a row without very good food options. You must try your best to figure out what happened and then do your best to make the changes needed to get back your momentum. Now let's talk about how your thoughts affect your losing weight.

Your reasons for wanting to lose weight in the first place may come into play when you notice that your momentum has gone down from where it was. Maybe you just wanted to see if you could do it—now that you have, the thrill is gone. Maybe there was a specific event and it has come and gone? Maybe it was to make that someone jealous and either you are back together now or have decided who cares? Regardless, it is time to take out your writing journal and look back to the beginning, and see why you wanted to lose weight in the first place. Does that reason still exist? How much did you want to lose? Are you close to it and maybe experiencing some sort of fear of success? Do you wonder: *What will I do after I lose the weight? Will I just gain it back again?*

There are many possible reasons that your mind can cause you to not be on your side in your journey to lose weight. The best thing to do is write down all the reasons you are making decisions that are *not in your best interest.* Just keep writing them until you no longer have any more thoughts as to why you are not going forward in your journey. Now look them over, and see which of them you would rate with an A as being a very likely problem, B as somewhat of problem, and then C as probably not really a problem at all. Tackle the A's and see what you can do about them, right now!! Here are *mine* from doing this exact exercise years ago:

» A–Too stressed—I feel the need to eat more often
» A–Too much work to do—Hard to find time to exercise
» B–Social Issues—I like going out for drinks and to eat with my friend
» B–Financial issues—Sometimes I am not able to sleep as well as I should
» C–Grocery shopping—So busy working, it is hard to find time to grocery shop

Let's go through these one by one and see what can be done:

A–Stress—Yes, I am stressed!!

- I could try to do certain stress reducing activities that I have already written down.
- I could eat pistachios when I feel stressed.
- I could get on the treadmill for 20 minutes (the amount of time it takes *me* to relieve stress by doing aerobic activity)

The last suggestion might be the best! But I love pistachios, so that is a good alternative when I can't workout. Truth be told, I really need to handle stress better, so getting out my list of stress reducing activities is a great idea—a massage, aromatherapy, or a heated neck roll (I am already starting to feel better; just thinking about my options)

A–Too much work to do—this is not a bad problem.

- Structuring my day could help—make a plan for my daily events and include a block of time or small blocks of time to workout
- Take breaks to workout for 10–20 minutes (small amounts of exercise are easier to fit into a busy day and combined make a good day's workout)
- Aerobics for 20 minutes
- Weights for 10 minutes
- Allow myself to work out an hour later than I used to—I used to workout no later than 6:00 pm, but I will try making 7:00 pm my cutoff time and see if it affects my sleep adversely or not. (It did not affect my sleep)

B–Social Issues—Yes, I like to go out with my friend, have a drink, and eat. But, we have been done it almost every night, lately. (Yes, I do get the irony that I am too busy, and I am still worrying about finances and I want to go out—however, he is also my business associate, so we do get a lot accomplished when we meet—though this may just be a rationalization!)

» The time and cost of doing this aside, where I eat and drink in and of itself does not prevent me from meeting my goals.
» I can choose the *best* option for food when we go out. I can put a little thought into it, and if my friend wants something different, I can evaluate whether it will work. If not, I can just say, "That sounds great, but maybe not tonight" and find a better solution that we are both happy with. I had an opportunity to try this shortly after making this list:

> *My friend and I were out for dinner and drinks that we were going to share when we had a dilemma—neither of us could agree on what to get. I wanted a fish entrée; he hates most cooked fish and wanted a burger and fries. I was not in the mood to be around french fries and not indulge. Then all of a sudden, we saw the cold seafood platter and found exactly what we both wanted. It turned out to be one of the most memorable evenings we had. Do not be afraid to work toward a mutual decision without making the other person responsible for your journey.*

So the social issues are really just a matter of choices to be made while we are out and not the actual activity of going out.

B–Financial Issues—we all have them, so it can hardly be an A and yet it is an issue I need to deal with, so it's not a C, either. It may begin to affect my sleep. I could:

» Go out to eat/drink less often

- Buy groceries that I know I will eat before they spoil
- See how far I have come in such a short amount of time and relax a little

I think that this aspect of my life is more in my control now than I give it credit for. Within a few short months of writing what I was sure to be my financial devastation, I completely restructured my finances. I brought in more business and diversified my practice into other areas that became even more rewarding both financially and intellectually. I have been able to set aside money in savings again, and turn my credit situation completely around. I surprisingly avoided the bankruptcy that I thought was imminent (through a twist of fate). I need to just get going with my life and not let the past financial issues worry me so much.

C–Grocery Shopping—being too busy to go to the grocery store could solve other problems such as spending money and being too busy, so I really don't see this as a problem. But, I wrote it down for a reason so I decided to look at why I wrote *grocery shopping* more closely.

- I go about once every other week, and a lot of stuff is frozen, so I have good choices available to me at all times with some effort
- But, I do not want or have the time to cook
- I could end up buying too much and letting it spoil if I went more often
- But, I do not always make good choices if my deli meats and produce are not fresh

So while I initially though this was a non-issue, I can see where going to the store more often and buying smaller quantities of fresh food would help me have better choices available to me when I am busy working.

Once I had gone through this list, there was something else I was feeling but didn't want to admit—I decided my biggest impediment to losing a little less than five pounds was writing this book. I decided to not continue writing and focused my efforts on myself. If and when I lost the weight, then I would decide if I even wanted to continue writing, since it seemed that finishing my book was stressing me out. I just went back to the basics—writing in my journal, making small-portioned meals, eating more often, and working out for about thirty minutes a day. The weight came off with very little effort and in very little time. And, of course I did decide to finish the book and share what I learned along the way. Our thoughts can have an enormous impact on our success, evaluating them is the best way to move forward.

Sometimes those last five pounds seem hard to lose; because you don't have the same incentive as you may have had when you first started your journey. It is easier to say, "Hey, I look pretty good—not exactly where I wanted, but good." This is where persevering and going forward is possibly harder than your earlier journey. If you find yourself at the point where you know you are making bad food choices for more than two days in a row, then stop for a moment and not only write down what and when you ate, but also why and how it made you feel at the time you ate and afterward. Only do this for a day or two. This introspection is critical to getting back on the path of meeting your goals.

There are some other things that can discourage you during the process. I will outline some of the most common discouragements and provide some ideas to help you move past them:

» ***It seems like I am throwing out food.*** This issue still affects me today, and I take as many precautions as I can to avoid letting food spoil. Just last week I opened up a brand new salad dressing from the refrigerator and found that the expiration date was six weeks ago! I haven't lived in the condo that long and I bought it after I moved in—probably two weeks ago. Clearly, I did not follow my own advice and look at the expiration date. So it made me wonder why? I think in this particular case, the dressing was on sale at half the original price. That is *not* a good reason to buy expired groceries. In retrospect, I think I failed to check the date, because the price was so low that I wanted to hurry up and buy it. Had I realized it was expired, I could have looked for one that was not; it wasn't the only one on sale! You may say, "How can the store sell perishable foods that are expired?" Human error! In a perfect world, you would not need to concern yourself with such matters—but you must!

Another reason for throwing out food is not planning your week properly. Eat your most perishable foods first—first fresh fish, second poultry, and third beef. Check your dates, and start to freeze if you aren't able to eat before the foods will no longer be fresh (before they are iffy!). Also, look ahead to see what days you may not even eat at home so you don't buy foods for days you have other plans. Or at the very least begin to select what you will freeze, if you realize you will not be eating at home as many nights as you first calculated.

» ***I am doing everything I am supposed to—yet I am still not losing weight.*** I want to be careful with this response, because there could be many issues at play here. Let's talk first about the areas that you need to make sure you have addressed as *everything* and then go from there:

  › Have you had your annual checkup? Did you get your blood work results and go over them with your doctor?

If not, go back and read over *Chapter 1—The Rules and Medical Stuff!*

- Are you getting 7–9 hours of sleep consistently?
- Are you under an unusual amount of stress recently?
- Are you exercising or engaging in some physical activity with movement *every* day for a minimum of 30 minutes?
- Are your food choices within reason that you don't feel guilty for what you ate?
- Are you eating till you are only satisfied, or have you allowed yourself to eat until you feel full, more often than not, recently?
- Are you eating before or as soon as you start to feel dizzy, hungry, or irritable? Or are you letting too much time pass between meals?
- Did you decide on your long-term goal? May be you were unable to set your final goal weight earlier in your journey—if yours has not been established—go for it and decide!!
- ***I was losing so much more weight each week compared to now.*** This is a little tricky in that it is true that not every week is the same, but you should make your goals based on what you have learned in *Chapter 5—How to Do It!* If you have made reasonable goals and are doing *everything* listed above, then address your goals and see if they are *your* goals or someone else's goals. Examine why you made the weekly goals you have. I truly believe that wanting something so badly is as important as all of the items above. If it turns out that the goals you made in the past are not yours—evaluate what goals you want and start from there.

Sometimes, you have to step back—especially if you have been on your journey for several months. It is possible for fatigue to set in. If you haven't taken a vacation from your routine, then go to *Chapter 8—Vacations and Business Travel* and give yourself permission to pretend you are on vacation for five to seven days. Pick the exact amount of time you will pretend you are on vacation, just as you would a real one, and then go back to your routine once those days are up. But, you must promise me you have had your annual checkup along with the proper blood work before, you take a vacation break due to lack of momentary motivation or momentum.

Since my last entry in this chapter nine months ago so much has changed...

For the most part, things were much better than they were the previous summer, when my business and finances were in complete chaos ... *until July 3, 2012;* when I got the call no parent ever thinks they will get. My oldest daughter, at age thirty-three, was hit by a car and instantaneously was gone; leaving behind her thirteen year-old son and husband of nine years and completely turning our worlds upside down.

When I said earlier, always be sure you can lose another five pounds if something unexpected happens. I did not think I would endure the exact thing I warned about. I lost over five pounds in less than two weeks. I was eating—but I lost weight nonetheless. I honestly did not care about my weight or myself—there were many more important things to focus on, like my grandson, my son-in-law, and my youngest daughter and her family. I miss my daughter every day...

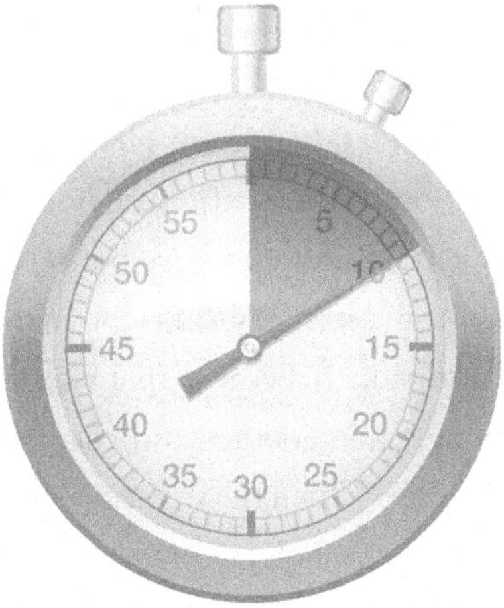

Chapter 7

Holidays and Various Events

You *can* keep your weight under control during the holidays and life's various events by making some simple changes in the way you approach them. Here are some tricks that I have used during the holidays and various events to help you along your journey.

Holidays

It is easy to gain weight during the holidays, especially during Thanksgiving, Christmas and other winter Holidays. But with a little forethought and a mind-set that you do *not* have to gain weight just because it is the holidays, you can make it through without affecting your waistline one iota. You will receive a lot of pressure to try everyone's cookies, fudge, and special drinks. Just make your own rules ahead of time, and stick to them (and have some handy excuses ready to deal with resistance).

Let's take a look at how you can make it through the holiday without adding extra weight in the process. Realize that going way off track can add up to five pounds in one day! I have done it (*many* years ago), and it is very sad—too many cookies, then a brownie; forget about eating lunch, because that was all in the morning. Co-workers brought homemade goodies and clients were having baskets delivered for the holidays! Then the sugar crash—the soda with caffeine to boost me up and then a holiday party. Nothing to eat at home, since there will be food at the party, right? This is the wrong way to think!

Eat your breakfast, lunch, and dinner! Each meal is very important, *especially* if you will be going to parties during the holidays. Breakfast will start your day off well-balanced and help you avoid the temptations at the office, like cookies or breads. If you do decide to have something you more than likely will eat a smaller amount since you have already had breakfast. Then at lunch have a lean-protein meal like grilled chicken or salmon on a bed of lettuce. During the holiday season when there are so many parties and goodies to choose from, it is important to eat more lean protein and fresh green vegetables when the menu options are in your control. There will be plenty of times when the menu is not in your control, and somehow, carbohydrate-rich foods end up at the party table. Be cautious, but always enjoy yourself!

So let's start with New Year's

If you are starting a weight loss program for the first time, New Year's Day is probably not the best day to start a weight loss program. Why? It will be considered a resolution, and most resolutions are not kept—so it's best not to put your journey into that category. If you are in the process of your journey and are continuing to lose weight, then decide what types of parties you will attend and what foods and drinks you will have to choose from. A party at your home allows for a lot of options that will satisfy you and let you enjoy the night. The following are appetizers and snacks to have out for that New Year's eve party that will keep you on your journey:

» Shrimp cocktail (Go easy on the cocktail sauce!)
» Mixed nuts
» Bacon-wrapped scallops
» Goat cheese and crackers
» Cheddar cheese and crackers
» Steak sliders

You want something that has more dietary fat and protein, if you will be drinking alcohol. While not all alcohol has carbohydrates in them, be sure to eat plenty of dietary fat and protein with your alcohol. New Year's Eve may be a good time to offer to be the designated driver and forgo the alcohol, at least until you are safely home.

Recipes with cream cheese are holiday favorites; however cream cheese has very little protein and a high amount of dietary fat; use Neufchâtel cheese instead.

If you attend a friend's party and it is appropriate to bring a dish, bring one that will provide you with the necessary nutrients to sustain you through the night. Bring enough, since it is possible your dish may be the one that everyone runs to. You don't want to eat the last bite of your own dish, so bring enough to share!

Super Bowl Sunday

This is really a national holiday, whether you like football or not. More than likely, you will be attending or preparing for a Super Bowl party. Even if you aren't asked, you can bring one or two menu items to ensure you have something you will feel good about eating. You can never have too much food at a Super Bowl party, but you can eat and/or drink too much—so pace yourself! Here are some menu ideas; if you are preparing for the occasion or attending a party:

» Wings (skip the dipping sauce—for yourself)
» Meatballs
» Chili and cheese with onions
» Tacos (homemade) with all the fixings
» Cheese and crackers platter
» Goat cheese on flavored crackers
» Stuffed cherry tomatoes
» Stuffed mushrooms
» Pigs in a blanket
» Ham with Neufchâtel cheese and green onions, rolled up
» Turkey and Swiss rolled up
» Deviled eggs (but only eat one!)
» Deli roast beef with horseradish cheese, rolled up
» Chicken nachos with cheese dip

Oh Valentine's Day!!

We may think of the obvious, like getting chocolates, but what about the dinner and soufflé with a bottle of champagne? Enjoy—but as always, do not overeat, and be sure to have dietary fat, protein, and carbohydrates included in your entire meal. Maybe start with oysters with champagne, or some Carpaccio with a glass of red wine, or some shellfish with a glass of white wine. You want to eat just enough to feel comfortable and be ready for whatever the night brings.

A favorite Valentine's Day food is chocolate-covered strawberries—if you are ready for dessert that is great. However, if you have not eaten a well-balanced meal already try something a little different. Maybe a cheese fondue with strawberries or artichoke hearts would be good. Or have a platter of bite size fruit and cheese cut into cubes already made up to feed each other. With a little planning and forethought, you can enjoy Valentine's Day with your loved one without making it into a restrictive night that is sure to put a damper on things. Remember *you* want to either maintain or lose weight—if your partner wants to indulge, so be it!

Memorial Day, 4th of July, and Labor Day

I lump these holidays together not because they are all patriotic holidays, but because they have a lot in common. They occur during the warmer months, outside activities are usually involved, lots of family and friends have their own ideas on foods to bring, there may be a barbeque, and there is a strong possibility of drinking!

If you have any say about the menu, go for almost anything grilled—steak, chicken, ribs, and most fish are amazing on the grill. I'm not against burgers and hotdogs. I am only against the large buns that usually go with them. Cut the bun in half and then cut the hot dog or burger in half and then double it on your bun. Twice the meat, half the bun, and easy on the condiments—but make sure you have enough to enjoy your meal.

For sides, have plenty of veggies without sauces; butter is fine. My favorite vegetables to have for barbeques are baked beans, green beans, and corn on the cob. For desserts, fresh fruit is the best, especially since it is in season. Watermelon or strawberries make great desserts during a holiday barbeque. If everyone wants something a little more traditional, try making homemade ice cream. Some of my favorite memories growing up during the summer were with my grandparents, making homemade ice cream. We had to hand-crank it, but it tasted amazing!

Halloween

Don't buy candy that you will want to eat yourself. There is usually some kind of candy that is not very tempting to you. For me, these candies are Almond Joy, Hot Tamales, and Gummy Bears—they just don't do it for me, so I feel very safe buying them. However, do not get me around a bag of Snickers, Reese's, or M&M's. I will eat them in a heartbeat! Keep this in mind when you pick up goodies to hand out. No one needs to know that you are not crazy about the candy you hand out. When there are leftovers, you won't be tempted to eat them, nor will you be tempted to open the bags ahead of time to get a taste.

If you have children and are used to getting into their candy, decide this year, it is hands-off! How much and how often you allow the kids to eat is a personal decision that you will need to make. If you can give some away to a good cause, do so. Some dentists have a program in which you bring in your Halloween candy and they donate it to the troops.

Thanksgiving

You may think, *I will eat what I want* or *I won't eat all day except Thanksgiving dinner.* Neither of these approaches will help you in the long run. How do you handle a day that is dedicated to nothing but eating? First, remember that Thanksgiving doesn't have to be anything more than a gathering of family and friends that includes dinner. That doesn't sound so ominous, does it?

Start your day like any other day—with a good breakfast that includes good sources of protein. My favorite Thanksgiving breakfast is bacon and eggs with a slice of toast with butter. If you are in weight loss mode, you may want to skip the toast. You will have plenty of breads and stuffing that day. Then do something to get your heart pumping; only five to ten minutes are needed. Calisthenics, brisk walking indoors or outdoors—start the day out feeling healthy and alive! Yes—sex counts! It's my favorite way to start out the holiday. Then go about preparing your Thanksgiving dinner as usual. There's no need to taste the food, since you already know what you are cooking, right?

Have some protein-rich foods out as appetizers. Then when it is time to eat, be sure to have a variety of foods that include vegetables—without sauces on them; butter is fine. Most likely your protein and will be turkey; but if you are one of the many who don't really care for turkey, be sure to have another source of protein at the table. Prime rib and ham are other traditional sources of protein, but feel free to have whatever you will want to eat! This is all assuming that you are hosting Thanksgiving dinner, which is not always the case.

One main reason we overeat at Thanksgiving is that we know it is a once a year event. Promise yourself that you will make a mini-Thanksgiving sometime again in the next couple of months. You can trade turkey for Cornish game hens and make all the fixings! If you happen to not get around to doing it, oh well! You have given yourself permission to do so, and you won't be as likely to overeat in the present!

In 2010, I attended two Thanksgiving dinners in the same day! I ate and drank alcohol at each one. My total weight gain for the entire week was 1½ pounds, which I promptly lost by the following Tuesday. I exercised in the morning and attended the first Thanksgiving at 1:00 pm, where I partook in the appetizers, entrée, and dessert along with a glass of wine or two! After helping with the cleanup of dinner I went for a walk with a friend. We just walked and talked for about 30 minutes—nothing strenuous. It was a great way to relax after all the hustle and bustle of the day as well as getting in some more exercise.

By about 5:00 pm, it was time to attend the next Thanksgiving dinner. This was close to three hours since the last time I ate and worked out perfectly! Once I got to the second Thanksgiving dinner, it was close to 6:00 pm before we ate, and I was ready to start all over again. But I did not overeat! I had a small portion of everything that I was interested in. You don't have to accept everything that is offered. Just politely say, "No thank you, not right now." I felt I needed a little more protein before having some pumpkin pie so I went back and had a little more of the turkey before dessert. The entire day I never felt stuffed!

If someone gives you a large piece of pie with whip cream this does not mean you have to eat it all! I promise—the host will get over it. If you ate every time someone made you feel guilty, that would be crazy! If all else fails and the host is insistent, offer to take your leftovers home, and then decide when you get home what to do with them. I think sometimes it is a generational thing for people to push more food on to others. When a polite, "No thank you" doesn't work, then say, "I would love more, but I can't right now. Would you mind boxing it up for me?" This puts it back on them to say yes or no. Usually, they will be glad to send you home with it. Who knows? Maybe they don't want it left in their house, either.

Christmas and Holiday Parties

There are many variations of Christmas and Holiday parties, and they each have their own issues; we will go over all the possibilities I can think of:

Evening Dinner including Appetizers, Dessert, and Alcohol

I recently attended one such event. While waiting for my cohort, I was in the bar, drinking water. I realized that I was 20 minutes early, and shortly we would have free food and alcohol, so why pay for it? I sat next to a lady who was discussing her struggle to lose 10 pounds and had offered to buy me a drink. I declined and then I realized that my decision to drink water at the bar while waiting for my friend to go into the main area for the party was really because I had ingrained into my head the need to eat when drinking alcohol and to not over-indulge too early in the night. About 15 minutes later she was getting ready to be seated with her guest asked again if I would accept her offer while I waited for my guest to arrive; I went ahead and accepted and had a glass of Prosecco. My friend arrived a few minutes later, and we went straight into the party, where I had two appetizers—bruschetta with cheese and a scallop wrapped in prosciutto—while I finished my Prosecco. Bruschetta with cheese would not have been my preference, but I was starting to get hungry and wasn't sure what other options I would have. I figured since there was some cheese included that it would be an okay choice. I was very glad when the scallops wrapped in prosciutto showed up. There were also crab cakes, but I passed on them. Crab cakes are not my favorite and are usually low in protein and high in dietary fat and carbohydrates.

But, let's digress a little to the beginning of the day and make sure we have brought up the obvious—you must eat throughout the day. The day began with breakfast including an egg. During the day there were well-balanced mini-meals after breakfast and then a moderately-sized meal about two hours prior to the party beginning.

Now that you are ready to attend your Christmas/Holiday party that includes appetizers, dinner, alcohol, and dessert—let's go through the main things to do and not do while you are at the party:

- Drink water when available —this may not be feasible to do until you sit down, when available alternate sips of alcohol and water.
- Select your appetizers carefully; there must be some protein in them, and ideally lots of it! Some good choices are
    - Shrimp cocktail (easy on the cocktail sauce)
    - Bacon-wrapped scallops

  - Pot stickers
  - Chicken skewers
  - Cheese cubes
  - Oysters
- If you are drinking alcohol, choose simple drinks and have no more than two drinks. Know your limits if you are driving. When you are losing weight, even two drinks can be too much!
  - Champagne or sparkling wine
  - Red or white wine
  - Martini without mixers
  - If you really want a holiday drink with eggnog, you will want to skip dessert!
  - Have some sparkling water with a twist of lime either as your main drink or an in-between drink as a way to feel a part of the festivities without the effects of the alcohol.
- Eat your salad, and skip the croutons. (You don't have to eat all of your salad.)
- Choose an entrée that is high in protein and easy on the starches. Avoid the pasta and avoid entrées with the words breaded, crusted, or fried. Some good choices are:
  - Fish
  - Chicken
  - Steak
  - Lamb
- Now for dessert—with a few exceptions, go for it! (Sometimes a few bites is very satisfying)
  - Did you drink your dessert? If so, then pass—say you are stuffed, even though you should not be stuffed; you should be satisfied.
  - Do you truly like the dessert being offered? If it is not

    - something that you would normally want, then don't eat it!
    - If you over did it during dinner, ate way too much, and really *are* stuffed—it can happen even with the best of intentions—then do not eat dessert!
- Especially if you are in weight loss mode, you may need to eat something before you go to sleep. This may seem odd; since you are positive you just ate a lot a few hours ago. If dinner was at 7:00 pm and you are ready to go to bed around 11:00 pm, that is enough time that you may want to have a couple pieces of cheese and crackers before heading off to bed.

That should take you through the traditional Christmas/Holiday parties. Let's look at the more casual office parties that are possibly at lunch or throughout the day in the office. These can actually be the most difficult!

Christmas or Holiday Party in the Office

Usually there are a lot of carbohydrates and fats at these events, so be careful! Sometimes these festivities are catered and other times they are potluck. Ironically, if they are potluck this may be your only fighting chance to have something at the party that is a good choice. As always, bring enough to share. Eat your breakfast as normal, and have a lean-protein morning snack. Deli meats like turkey or chicken are good choices—add a cracker for some crunch. As you look at your options at the office party, choose items that you feel will be well-balanced as your main choices. Feel free to have some of the other goodies, but keep it to two bites of each item. This may seem like it is not enough, but you want to remember your goals and how far you have come. Is it worth it to give up all that progress just to indulge yourself rather than having just a taste? If you really don't think you can help yourself from eating too much, then just don't go. Maybe you have an appointment that came up unexpectedly.

Your Own Office during the Holidays

Sometimes our own office can be more difficult to navigate the social protocol and the guilt and/or desire to try everything, nothing, or just what you are interested in. Your best defense at this time of the year is to come up with your own rules! If you happen to know that your biggest client always sends cookies or brownies, you may want to allow yourself to have one cookie or half a brownie on the day it arrives—besides, the first day *is* the best day. You could make a rule that if the food is more than a day old, you won't eat it. Either before or shortly after you have the goody; eat something with protein in it. If you don't already, be sure to have cheese sticks, beef jerky, or nuts available in your office so you have a quick mini-meal at your fingertips.

What about co-workers who bring all the goodies they baked to share? Again, before the holidays get underway, think about how you want to handle these issues. Say to yourself ahead of time, "If this item comes along, I will have *some*, and if these others come along, I don't want them." You will keep the desires at bay by deciding ahead of time what and how much you are going to eat! You may say a two-inch square cookie is good. If one comes in that is four inches, you will only eat half!

These are your rules, so think carefully about them, and decide on what will make you happy and what is just not worth it! When your co-workers' ask if you tried their goody that was not on your list, just say, "No, I haven't tried it yet." Soon enough, they will be eaten up by everyone else, and the issue will be moot! You may want to scream, "No! Don't you know I am trying to lose weight?" Don't do it. It won't make you feel any better. Then they will try to tell you, "It's just *one;*

it won't hurt you." Or worse, the next goody that is brought in *is* on your list of okay items. Then if you eat that goody people are going to wonder if you gave up on losing weight, didn't like them or the goody that you wouldn't eat the other day—just don't go there.

Baking for School and Other Functions

Sometimes you just have to bake for the kid's school function or some other reason. You may wonder: *How will I do this without wanting to eat some myself.* If it is possible to make something that you cannot cut into without being noticed, that would be ideal. Brownies, fudge, a cake, baked bread, or pies are great options. You can pack them up and send them off without even concerning yourself with eating them. If you need to make cookies or cupcakes that would be easy for you to take without being noticed; decide ahead of time if you are going to allow yourself to have one. If you have decided that it is okay for you to do so, eat something with protein before you start baking. Then enjoy your baked goodies guilt-free, and stick to the amount that you decided on.

If you decide that it is *not in your best interest* to have one of your baked goodies at this time, bake with others around, including your kids. It is a great lesson to teach them that when you cook and/or bake, you do not need to eat or taste everything. My grandmother instilled that in us as young children. We were not allowed to lick the beaters, taste our food, or eat our baked goods until the appropriate time (after dinner). When I got older, I decided that it was really yummy to eat my baked goods as they came out of the oven and over did it! Now I know why my grandmother said not to do it.

After the baked goods are cooled off, box them up, and seal them so that you are not tempted to get into them before they are sent off to school. You can even use ribbons, bows, stickers—anything that would give you a second to think, *do I really want to do this?*

If all this seems like torture, just remember that if you were buying a friend's birthday present, you wouldn't feel like you were being tortured if you didn't buy yourself the exact same thing! You are creating a gift for others, so take pride in your gift, and continue on your journey.

Coffee, Creamers, Cocoa, and Eggnog, etc.

During the holidays, beverages are just as much a part of the season as the foods. Whether it is of the alcohol nature or not, these beverages can add inches to your waistline in the blink of an eye.

> *Make your beverage decisions as carefully as you make your food choices, and continue to include water in between your holiday beverages.*

Normally, coffee would not be a concern, but during the holidays, sugared creamers are the mainstay everywhere I look—pumpkin spice, peppermint mocha, and eggnog. These are loaded with sugar. I am not saying to not have any, just remember to offset your coffee with protein and some dietary fat—a cheese stick or some nuts. It is best to have one coffee with flavored creamer and then go back to half and half. If you can get flavored coffee beans, this is your best option. My favorite is amaretto or hazelnut; flavored coffee beans normally do not add any calories to the coffee. When I want a little holiday flair to my coffee I add cinnamon chips.

Hot cocoa with whipped cream or marshmallows is another holiday favorite. If you can make your whipped cream from scratch with a beater, this is best. Or just enjoy the cocoa by itself, and skip the toppings altogether. The best cocoa uses whole milk and real melted cocoa—the less processing, the better.

Buy your favorite brand of eggnog, and enjoy *some;* go all out, and get the expensive gourmet kind. Whatever you do, do *not* get the low-fat kind—it will not taste as good, will have more carbohydrates, and will not be as satisfying. On the first holiday right after my weight loss journey, I decided not to have any eggnog, since I wasn't sure if I could only have one glass. I decided cold turkey was better for me at the time, but now having been in maintenance mode for a while, I feel comfortable having a glass or two during the holidays. I make sure to not keep it in my house. I pick it up on the way to someone else's house (along with some amaretto), and then I leave it there!

Apple cider is a little deceptive, since it is seems like a healthy alternative to the other holiday drinks. It is not that it is *not* healthy; it is that cider is almost all carbohydrates. Therefore, you would need to eat something with protein and some dietary fat; which if you were only planning on having something to drink, will add unneeded eating to your holidays.

Holidays in Summary

My hope is that you come to enjoy the holidays for what they were meant to be—time to spend with family and friends—and not just another diversion in your weight loss journey or worse gatherings that reverse all the progress you have made thus far! Celebrating the holidays is no longer a foregone conclusion that you will gain weight.

Various Events

Having your menus made up ahead of time and relying on them will keep the following kinds of events from derailing you! If you do not have a plan for these occasions, they will become a problem for you!

Visiting Other People's Offices

Sometimes you need to be out of your environment; where you may not have much control over your time table. Such is the situation when you are in someone else's office for an extended period of time. Anything over two hours where you are unable to eat at will, you need to make sure you have eaten a well-balanced meal within an hour before the meeting—one hour prior should allow for driving time to the meeting. If this is not the case, plan to eat at a restaurant close by prior to your business meeting.

Bring your own cold water (in case there is none available) and individual packages of nuts or a cheese stick in your purse. If needed, step into the bathroom and have a bite or two. (Keep textured teeth wipes in your purse so no one knows you just ate anything!) This can all be done in 60 seconds if needed. The other option is to make it through the meeting and eat when you get into your car. You will be prepared, and you won't be so ravenous that you just stop anywhere close by to eat *something.*

If your meeting is early in the morning, be sure to eat something with eggs in it beforehand, even if you aren't particularly hungry. Sometimes when you have to wake up earlier than you are used to, your body just isn't hungry yet, but you still need to eat your breakfast before you head out or while you are on the way to the appointment.

Conferences

When you attend a conference, you have a couple of factors to concern yourself with. The most important is staying alert and attentive to what you are there to learn. The second issue is that the breaks and foods available (or not available) are pretty much out of your control. Be prepared!

You want something that isn't noisy, and nuts are probably the noisiest snack, so only eat them while you are on break so as not to disturb others. A good option during the conference is beef jerky (only the tenderloin chunks); it is lightly chewy and shouldn't bother others. I also like to bring cheese sticks, but I have them in the early hours of the conference so they are eaten within 2–3 hours of being put in my purse. I also recently figured out how to travel with cheese sticks by packing them with an ice-pack and then keeping them in the room with the ice bucket—saving time looking for cheese when I get to the hotel. I know these options are not many, and I continue to look for foods to bring to a conference keeping in mind both the ease of obtaining (gift shops or prepackaging), ease of eating without disturbing others, and have them be foods that will help keep you alert!

If there ever was a time to stay away from the soda, it is at a conference! Stick to coffee with cream (but no sugar) and lots of water! Do not eat any sweets at break time! There is no protein to counteract the sugar during a break; this will turn into a disaster for your conference. You will be inattentive, dizzy, and possibly fall asleep—oh yes it happens! At a conference, lunch or dinner is the time to have dessert if you would like something sweet—limit your carbohydrates during your meal; and do not eat the entire dessert.

Breakfast is probably something you do not think about when at a conference. Some conferences offer a continental breakfast; which is primarily carbohydrates. Continental breakfasts do include fruit, but remember—fruits are carbs! Bring your own cheese stick or cottage cheese (from the diner) to add to the fruit and you will have a well-balanced breakfast. Some of the better conference breakfasts include cottage cheese and/or hard-boiled eggs. Unless you are absolutely sure there will be good sources of protein provided at the conference breakfast, allow time to eat a substantial breakfast before you attend. Omelets, bacon and eggs, or cottage cheese with a slice of fruit are all great options.

Shopping

When planning a couple hours or more of shopping, think about your dining options; bring water and cheese sticks that you can keep in your purse. When you are shopping, you do not want to make bad choices only because you want to continue shopping but have gotten hungry or feel dizzy. Being thirsty may make you feel like you are hungry, so always bring cold water with you when shopping.

Shopping is probably one of my favorite workouts. Trying on clothes, carrying bags, and all that walking does count! Cheese sticks are easy to eat on the run while walking from one store to the next, and even if there isn't any place to throw out your wrapping, you can stick it back in your purse till later without making a mess. The other good thing is that there is very little chance of getting your hands dirty while eating.

If you need to have a meal, know your food court, and seek out choices that will keep you going and not weigh you down. My favorite is half a tuna sandwich on sourdough with a small salad, and I skip the cookie. Drink water with your meal to keep hydrated while shopping.

Movies

Who doesn't love to go to the movies and get a bucket of popcorn and large soft drink? Surprisingly not everyone—you may do this because of habit rather than real desire, so think about it and see if you really want to continue this tradition—maybe you can make a new one. If you feel you truly need to keep *this* particular tradition and you do not go to the movies very often, say 2–3 times a year, then have a small bag of popcorn with butter and try to skip the soft drink. Once you have given up soda you will realize you do not need to have it in order to do the normal things you once did when you drank soda.

If you happen to go to the movies a lot and want to continue doing so and not feel left out of the normal routine, there are a few ways around this: (1) have a small amount of popcorn (do *not* eat out of the bag—see if you can get a separate bag for the amount you selected, bring your own paper bag, or put it in a napkin), (2) every other time you go you will have some, (3) use the game of picking a number between 0–9 and if the day you are going to the movie has that number then you will have some, (4) have two bites of something that someone else gets, or (5) you can decide that it is just *not in your best interest* to eat any of the movie foods. Eat a satisfying, well-balanced meal beforehand, regardless of your decision.

It may seem like *everybody* gets popcorn, a large soda, and a jumbo-sized candy at the theater, but they don't. If you can get to the point where you don't feel like you are depriving yourself by not partaking in this perceived ritual, you will allow yourself to enjoy the movie without the trappings!

There are now more movie theatres being built or retrofitted to serve real meals as part of the movie experience. Know your menu options before you get to the theater, they are just like restaurants—there are good choices if you look.

Moving

I recently moved and found this process to create some craziness I did not anticipate with regard to eating right and working out. It took almost two months to complete the move. I had 20 years of memories I had to process and the house I was moving from required construction before I could put it up for sale. I continually found myself driving to the old house before the crack of dawn to let contractors in. Moving presented a new set of issues when it came to maintaining my weight.

Breakfast is a must! The tried-and-true breakfast of an egg over easy with some meat and a slice of toast is great, but if you are on the move (so to speak), stop by a place that has an egg breakfast sandwich. (Check online for the best food options to start off your day.)

Always weigh yourself in the morning right after waking up just to make sure everything is okay and you are on top of the situation. If you can write down or text yourself what you eat, that is great! If not, then stick to the basics. Remember to eat every two to four hours. Have some easy-to-eat foods in the refrigerator:

- » Crackers and pepper turkey
- » Goat cheese and crackers
- » Hard boiled Eggs with cherry tomatoes
- » Deli roast beef and Swiss cheese
- » Cottage Cheese and bananas

In the freezer, keep some TV dinner entrées (preservative free is the best). You don't need to eat the whole entrée. You can always retrofit a TV dinner by taking out *some* of the pasta or rice and tossing them before you start to eat. When cooking is not an option, a good TV dinner will keep you going!

Bonus: If you are doing some of the lifting and carrying during the move, then you do not need to work out! Lift the boxes you can reasonably lift, and walk them downstairs (if you feel you are coordinated enough). Always lift and walk responsibly, wear a good pair of tennis shoes, and you will have no problem keeping to your routine and getting a great workout in the process. Remember to stretch!

It is very tempting to order pizza and beer—I get it! It took me two months to move. One night, I said, "I want pizza and red wine." I knew I should get something else to round it out, so I got wings along with the pizza. It was delicious, I won't lie, but I also gained 2½ pounds within 24 hours. (I had the pizza and wings for breakfast, lunch, and the next dinner.) You need to decide if it is worth it. I could have had the pizza and wings for just one night, and that probably would have set me back less than I gained by eating it for all of my meals. The reason I ate it for all of my meals was because I knew I rarely if ever order pizza, so I thought I really needed to take advantage of this opportunity. I'm only human!

Sporting Events

I *love* going to sporting events! But finding food there; well somehow I ended up with a soft pretzel, and then I started adding cheese to it so I felt like it was more balanced, or I get cotton candy or birthday cake ice cream along with a hot dog—of course to add some balance! Besides what else was I supposed to eat, I was at a sporting event! I decided to take a stand back and really look to see what there really was to eat. I was surprised to find the following choices at a recent football game in the main concourse:

- Cheeseburger (no fries)
- Cinnamon Almonds/Pecans
- Chicken Tenders without sauce
- Hot Dog with half the bun
- Chili and Cheese w/onions
- Chicken Breast Sandwich
- Pulled Pork Sandwich
- Peanuts and Almonds

I chose the cheeseburger and used the *fake bun eating method* (that is where each bite you take you are really only eating the meat patty and the bottom bun—while still holding onto the entire burger—you keep pushing the bottom bun and patty up for the next bite). The alcohol selection in the main level was very small. The choices were all kinds of beer, Mike's Hard Lemonade, and a freshly made margarita. My personal choice at a sporting event is a bloody Mary, if available. Water is sometimes the best option.

Normally there is not a lot of exercising while sitting at a sporting event. However, if you have a chance to walk a little farther for parking or take the stairs a few more times, go for it! Always think of safety when deciding to take stairs or walk farther in a parking lot; but there is usually a lot of security at sporting events. When there are breaks in the game think about walking inside the stadium until you find a bathroom that doesn't have a line, rather than standing *in* line.

Treat these days like any other. Weigh yourself when you wake up, make a well-balanced breakfast, and time your meals so that you eat about 1½–2 hours before you arrive at the sporting event. If you want to drink alcohol, keep it to one or two drinks, and alternate with water. As always know your limits when you are losing weight, when it comes to alcohol, a little can go a long way. Then when you get back home, keep on track with a good dinner, including a lean protein and some veggies! If when you get back it is already time for bed, and are hungry, have some cheese and crackers.

Skiing or Other Winter Sporting Activities

When you need something to take the edge off and keep you going, there is nothing better than a cheese stick. You can put it in a pocket or bag, and it is good for quite a while on the slopes. If you ski, one of these cheese sticks can mean the difference between having to get off the slopes and continuing on. If you decide to get off the slopes for some much needed nourishment, the best option is chili with cheese. Most ski lodges will have this as an option, and it provides a great combination of dietary fat, protein, and carbohydrates!

Skip the alcohol while on the slopes. It is best to not drink alcohol while skiing for a couple of reasons. Skiing requires you to be alert *and* you are on your weight loss journey; it is possible that the effects of alcohol combined with the altitude may not be what you are used to. If you want to partake in alcohol, do so at the end of the day when you are safely in your lodge!

Lake or Water Sporting Activities

An ice chest, even a small one will allow you to have cold water and some fresh fruit and cheese while you are on a boat or lakeside. Grapes are the best fruit and cheese cubes in a bag. Beef jerky is always a hit with the kids when they have been on the lake wake boarding! All of these are easy to eat and do not create much litter (always keep your litter in the ice chest until you can put it in the trash). Water sports and boating do not mix well with alcohol and can be very dangerous—wait until you are on dry land.

Hiking

Have twice the water you think you will need. Use a backpack that holds water allowing constant access to it. There should also be a place to put some snacks—smoked almonds are best—they will not make as much of a mess as other seasoned almonds. Avoid trail mix that you will need to sift through and decide what and what not to eat (never drop or leave food on a hiking trail; if you want to bring trail mix sort through it at home so that you can eat whatever is left).

Golf

It may be tempting to wait for that drink cart to come around, but more than likely, it will *not be in your best interest*. Stay focused on your game, drink only water, and bring along some pre-shelled pistachios, cashews or unseasoned almonds (less messy) in a closeable bag. The sun mixed with alcohol is a bad combination and could not only dehydrate you and wreak havoc with your game; it may cause you to eat anything on that drink cart! Your better option is to wait until you get to the clubhouse—then combine a well-balanced appetizer or meal with your alcohol if you still wish to partake in the libations!

What if you are at a golf tournament or social game where drinking is a given? Be sure to eat a mini-meal that is moderate in carbohydrates and higher in dietary fat and protein right before you go, and keep some almonds on hand to snack on when needed. Keep water on hand as well. Switch back and forth between the water and the alcohol. This will help keep you hydrated and lessen the effects of the alcohol on you and your game!

Musicals

The options available to eat and drink surprised me when I went to a musical. They caught me off guard, and I ended up eating the most amazingly soft and yummy cookies! I also did not feel so well after eating them, either. Let's start at the beginning.

My family debated whether to meet for dinner prior to the musical. I could have made a good dinner for myself around 5:30 pm, but I *didn't*. I thought there would be some good food options since it was held at a very nice auditorium—and I was right. I started with a chicken Caesar salad and a glass of cabernet (so far so good). But, then my sister wanted some cookies and asked if I would wait in line and get some for her (*that* I was not expecting—I had stayed away from the desserts on purpose). There were many options, and I had no idea which ones she would like. I knew which ones I would like, and I proceeded to buy two bags of freshly-made cookies. (There were three cookies in each bag.)

I *knew* I didn't need them—especially since I had a glass of wine—but I didn't think about it ahead of time. I just figured, *it's a Christmas musical, so I can eat sweets, and besides I am maintaining, and how often do I really get out like this?* All the rationalizations came to me at once. I ate two of the cookies and put the last one in my purse and then later the trash (after offering it to everyone else). Think ahead!

Sick Time

You may actually gain weight eating chicken noodle soup and crackers and drinking ginger ale or lemon-lime soda. Do not despair. Once you have eaten one day's worth of real food and not sick people food, you can resume exercise in basic beginner mode at 10–15 minutes of cardio per day. Do some light walking, and do not lift weights. Increase very gradually each day based on how you feel. I recommend working out at home until you are able to workout for at least 30 minutes at a time. You should be up to your normal workout routine *no sooner* than one week and no later than two weeks. *Stop* immediately if you feel dizzy or tired. You may have started too soon. Sometimes taking one more day of rest is the best thing to do rather than worry about your weight.

Do not overeat or drink too much ginger ale or lemon-lime soda while you are sick. Sip, sip, sip, and you will get through this sick time and get back on track as soon as you feel better. If you happen to lose weight, you are probably going to bounce back some, so don't get discouraged if you lose a few pounds and then gain a couple back when you start eating normally. Just be sure that you ease back into normal eating. Start out by eating half of what you would normally eat before you were sick—your stomach may have shrunk, if you lost weight while you were sick. If you are still hungry, try to wait an hour, and have a little more food. Remember to go back to your menus, and see what sounds good.

If you were sick for more than a couple of days, the food in your refrigerator may have gone bad. If you thought to freeze any of the meats once it became apparent you were not going to eat them—that is great! Do not beat yourself up if you didn't—life happens! This is when having canned and frozen foods will come in handy, since your first thought once you start to feel better will not be, *let's go grocery shopping!* It will be: *I am hungry!* Once you feel better take an assessment of your refrigerator, decide what is still good and what is not, and toss the bad food!

Pregnancy

Go to your doctor as soon as you think or know you are pregnant!

- *Ask how much your doctor believes you should gain right up front*—and schedule out a time frame for approximate weight gain for each phase of the pregnancy
    - Do not obsess about your weight gain; your doctor really is the best person to talk to about what is best for you!!
    - Do not use this time as a *reason* to eat anything and everything to excess—you should not overeat during anytime in your life.
- *Ask your doctor what foods and drinks are off limits*—during each phase of your pregnancy and post pregnancy—specifically if breastfeeding
    - Check each time you are pregnant—medical science advances and each pregnancy is different. What may be deemed not harmful during your first pregnancy may now be considered unsafe during your second and visa-versa.

- *Ask your doctor how much exercise is okay for* ***you***—during each phase of your pregnancy.
  - Find out which exercises you should avoid and which are recommended while you are pregnant—again, check each time you are pregnant—each pregnancy is different.
  - Knowing which exercises *you* should do will depend greatly on what you were doing right before you got pregnant—so be sure to let your doctor know what your exercise routine was for the three months prior to becoming pregnant.
- Ask your doctor about your post-pregnancy workouts *before* you deliver
  - Ask your doctor when you can start working out and what exactly you can do post-pregnancy. The answer will depend on your delivery. You may not see your doctor for a few weeks after the delivery—so if the delivery goes a little different than expected—you will want to get an update on your post-pregnancy plan before you leave the hospital from your doctor.
  - The easiest time to lose weight after your pregnancy is during the three months after you deliver, so take advantage of this window of opportunity while adhering to your doctor's orders!

No Time to Make Anything

You may wonder, *how this is an event?* But it may be the *one* event that will get you off course, the fastest! Your menus will be of the utmost importance here; you will need to quickly assess the situation. Is it that you have no time to make something, no time to eat something, or no time for either?

- Can you cook while you do whatever issue is pressing?
- Can you eat something while doing something else?
- Do you need to make *and* eat something quickly?

Here are some ways to resolve the above issues:

- Have something cooking while continuing to work and then stop and eat for a few minutes. Baked or microwave dinners are perfect in this case—retrofit a TV dinner by removing some of the rice or pasta, if needed, to reduce the carbohydrates.
- If you have a few minutes to make something, go to your five minutes or less meals and select from there. Maybe a sandwich or cottage cheese with fruit—something that you can eat while working and not spend too much time preparing.
- If you do not have anytime at all and need to eat immediately, then eat one of the one minute or less items from your menus—a hard-boiled egg, some nuts, a slice of cheese, or some deli meat with a bite or two of fresh fruit (grapes or berries are easy to eat when short on time)

Physical Injury

Physical injury has the potential to derail you during your weight loss journey. I suffered an *acute* ankle injury (from tripping while walking into a ballroom at a conference I was attending) four months into my weight loss journey—my goal was only seven weeks away. I could have given up or delayed my goal; no one would have known but me—and even if I had let others know about my goal, I am sure no one would have held it against me if I decided to delay my goal due to my injury. But I felt I had momentum and I was on target to reach my goal by my birthday. I decided to look at my exercise program and see what changes I could make once I took a week to recuperate to the point I could walk without assistance for a reasonable amount of time.

The first change I obviously had to make was not using my treadmill, elliptical, or leg presses. I could, however, do leg exercises while lying on the floor without any weights, including inner thighs and outer thighs—so this seemed promising. I was also able to resume using my recumbent bike at the easiest resistance. I decided to add one pound arm weights to the time I was on the bike to do double duty while in recovery. The only change I made to my eating was to be vigilant about eating when I started to feel hungry, only eating till satisfied, and not let myself get dizzy or eating as soon as I was.

So that is what I did for the remainder of my six weeks for exercise—I reached my goal by my 47th birthday of 130.0 pounds!! About a month later I was able to start using the treadmill and elliptical again. I am *very* glad that I did not give up when I hurt my ankle. I would hate to wonder what would have happened had I done so.

Various Events in Summary

There are a lot of events that will happen that can get you off course. Deal with each of them as they occur. If you feel you didn't handle them so well the first time, learn from the experience and remember to enjoy the journey.

Have you gone on a vacation lately? Are you planning one? I have great news; there is a whole new way to handle your weight loss journey while on vacation that you are sure to enjoy! So let's go to—*Vacations and Business Travel.*

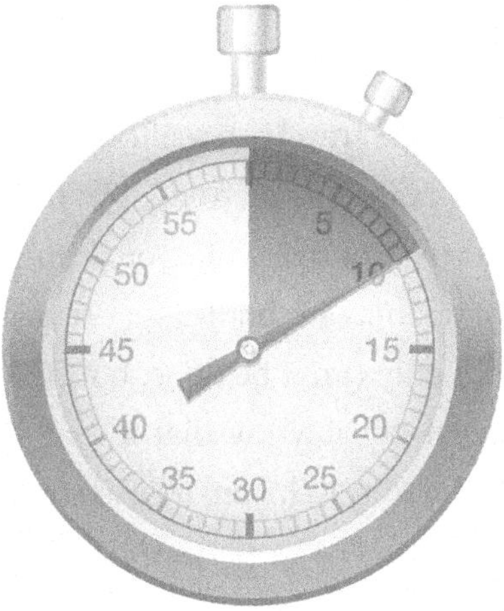

Chapter 8

Vacations and Business Travel

Vacations are different from business travel, but they have the same issues. *You are away from your home for an extended period of time and at the mercy of your environment. You also must be able to make quick decisions based on little forethought.* It is possible that you may gain *some* weight (not more than your *never again* number), but there are ways to safely lose it as soon as possible and get back on track as soon as you get home!

Let's first examine the differences business travel and personal travel. If you are on personal travel, then you are on vacation and taking a hiatus from writing in your journal and weighing in every day. If you are a business traveler, then there's no such luck; you are still writing in your journal and you will be checking on your midsection measurements every morning.

Business Travel

Business travel can seem to wreak havoc with your weight loss journey, but I caution you to not use this as a reason for not keeping with your normal routine while you are out of town. I have seen many people who have amazing bodies that travel for work the majority of the time; so not only can it be done, but business travelers may have it easier. How can I possibly say that it may be easier? I found that when I am on business travel, I am focused on my work and not on eating or drinking. Sometimes I work during dinner and either skip the drink or only have one since I have so much work to do in such a short time period. I also have some freedom to be in charge of my time, with the exception of a few conferences that others initiate.

You travel for a purpose—to close a deal, make another sale, or work on a business issue—so use this diversion to your advantage. If your business travel doesn't consume your evenings, bring projects that will keep you engaged and not thinking about drinking a bottle of wine at the local bar along with a full five-course meal. This can be tempting if the company is paying for it! If you do need to entertain clients while out of town, just treat it like any other dinner in town. Do not overeat—eat a well-balance meal, don't overdo the alcohol, and if you can fit in a 15–30 minute walk before or afterward, that is even better.

Most hotels have fitness centers and indoor or outdoor swimming pools that can be used year-round—ask for the available times when you check-in. Within minutes, you are at a gym. If there is no fitness center in your hotel, bring your own! Flexible bands are the best for resistance training and take up virtually no space in your luggage. Don't forget your sneakers, and get some walking in. If you have the opportunity to walk barefoot along the beach, that is the best. Enjoying the sunrise or sunset along the beach is amazing and walking barefoot in the sand is great for your calf muscles. If you do *not* know the area or have any weather concerns, do not go where you do not feel comfortable. The best thing to do in this case is walk throughout the hotel. You can do this in heels if you forgot your tennis shoes.

If you go on vacation a lot—you will want to follow this advice as well—bring a small, soft tape measure with you while you travel. Two days before you leave town, measure your midsection as soon as you wake up (this is the area below your belly button and above your hips). Continue to weigh yourself in the morning. Write your weight and measurement in your journal and on a piece of paper. Put the piece of paper in your luggage, and then while you travel, measure your midsection every morning. Make adjustments to what or how much you eat and how often you exercise if you find your midsection increasing.

The vacation section has valuable information for business travelers as well. The section *Problems Which May Occur* and below includes advise for both business travelers and vacationers.

Vacations

While you are on vacation, there is no need to weigh yourself every day—or at all, for that matter! If there is a scale in your room, it will not be the same as the one at home, so either it will give you a false sense of security or make you feel bad about yourself. Neither is what you want to feel while on vacation. I don't even weigh myself at home on the day I fly out, especially if I fly out in the morning!

If you vacation less than three weeks per year, then you can take your measurement before you leave town if you want. Tuck it away in your luggage just in case you are worried that you will gain weight—but it isn't necessary. If you really want to weigh yourself to keep on track, get on the scale in the morning after you have gotten one full night's sleep. Do not freak out *or* get excited about the number; it is only your baseline number to compare to following days when you choose to weigh yourself in the morning. Decide the first time you get on the scale how much weight gain is acceptable; my recommendation is about three pounds. If you are close to gaining three pounds, then reassess how much you eat at each meal. Be sure you are not overeating. Gaining weight while you are on vacation should not spell disaster for your plans, self-esteem, or ability to lose the small amount that you gained as soon as you are home.

Enjoy the Cuisine—without Overeating

The thing that will be the hardest to do while on vacation is to *not* overeat. One of the main reasons for overeating is due to a feeling of scarcity or not being able to eat this particular food again, if only for a while. This usually is not true, but on vacation, it may be true! You must be ready for the reality that you will come across a meal that will be amazing! Remind yourself that the meal will be more memorable if you eat a reasonable portion and don't over-indulge to the point that you have painfully overeaten. Think of a time when you overate and how you felt awful—think about this before you even go to the restaurant so when that amazing meal does come, your mind will help you eat a reasonable portion. If it is possible and others agree, decide while you are there to come back for another meal at this amazing place while you are on vacation. This will help relieve the feeling of never getting to eat there again!

Be sure to enjoy the local cuisine. Try letting someone else who knows the area or restaurant pick out your meals. It can be very liberating! Always retain veto power, but it can be fun to try something that you have never tried before. Try anything and everything that appeals to you. In my city of Phoenix, the rattlesnake is quite the indigenous cuisine. If I were to say while on vacation, all fried foods are off-limits, then I would not be able to eat it, since it is almost always served fried. This rule would keep me from enjoying my vacation. Try to not have so many rules while on vacation.

> *Several years ago I went on a cruise with my entire family, and there were a few friends of our family as well. The first night one of the friends announced that he had decided to stop drinking—that day—the first day of the cruise. (A worthy thing to do...) except, he was only doing it so he would not gain weight on the cruise. Well, within less than 24 hours his resolution was over.*

The first day of your vacation is not the time to start putting new rules in place—enjoy your vacation and be reasonable in your selections and when you can't; be even more reasonable in your quantities.

Exercising When Out-of-town

While you are on vacation, you should get some good old-fashioned walking in. Vacations can provide great built-in exercise regimens. Take the stairs if that is an option; remember to always be safe. Walk with others and only in areas that your hotel recommends or that you are familiar with. The best way to enjoy your vacation guilt-free is to include a fair amount of exercise to offset the indulgence in the local fare and the libations that are part of any great vacation.

However, your vacation may not include ample time to walk or hike. You may spend time on the beach, lying down and not playing volleyball or Frisbee. You may be on a boat and not water skiing or swimming. You have a couple of options. You can forget about it and just relax *or* go to the fitness center at your hotel and workout vigorously for no more than 20 minutes. *Why only 20 minutes—because, you are on vacation!* Get some cardio in, like an elliptical or stair stepper, and then do some arm weights—do a few triceps and biceps, and then head back to the fun!

Business Travelers and Vacationers

Problems Which May Occur

Another problem that can occur while away from home is what I call, *vacation constipation*. Sometimes it seems a little more difficult to be regular while out of town, whether by yourself or with others. The lack of familiarity and the additional people in a smaller space can make your bowels a little shy! This is very common and may not be entirely avoided. Try to get up early enough to allow time to use your own bathroom before heading out, if possible. You may need to wake up even earlier if you share a room with multiple people.

If coffee is part of your normal routine, be sure to either make coffee in the room when you wake up or have it preordered so that it arrives at the same time you wake up. This will help you keep with your normal routine. At the very least, drink a glass of water upon waking if you aren't able to get your coffee fix in.

Give yourself permission to go in a public restroom. Some people are a little more than bowel shy, and the thought of doing a number two where someone else can hear them just doesn't seem right. Get over it! You do not know any of these people, and if you do know them, they are friends and family who are dealing with the same issues. They may actually be relieved to know it's not just happening to them. If the moment arises and it's time to go—just go. You will feel much better once you do!

The Minibar

You can make your own rules; just remember to make them ahead of time so that you are not caught off guard when the minibar invites you. You can also decline the key when you check in. Just know that there are good options, okay options, and options that are *not in your best interest.*

Coming Back Home

You did your best—or maybe not. You are back from vacation, and it is time to get back on track. *Do* not *weigh yourself as soon as you get home!* It is tempting to see how much you gained, but resist the temptation. Have one full night of sleep at home, and then get on the scale in the morning once you have voided your bladder. The best thing you can do on your first day back is get a good night's sleep—at least eight hours. If you are truly exhausted and dealing with jet lag then no more than 11 hours. I always make it a point to get on the time zone that I am in the first night. This may mean I go to bed earlier or later than I usually would. If you are able to adjust to the time zone you are in the first night, you will get back into your routine much faster.

I am sure you are wondering why I am so adamant about not weighing yourself until after you have had a good nights sleep. There are a few reasons: (1) it just doesn't matter what you weigh during the day or night time; the only weight that matters is what you weigh in the morning, (2) you may be discouraged to find that you gained five pounds or more; which if you weigh yourself later in the day, is very possible, and (3) if you are discouraged, you may think, *what the heck I will just eat whatever I want tonight. I've already gained too much weight, so why try to eat normally yet?* That is exactly the wrong attitude; get back into your normal eating *as soon* as you get home.

There are different ways to return to your journey—based on what time of day you return. If you get back earlier in the day, begin eating smaller meals (about half of what you normally would eat) every 1½–2 hours. Be sure to set your timer for two hours, since your schedule and appetite will probably not be quite back to normal yet. Start recording everything in your journals again as soon as you get home. You may need to cut the blocks in your journal in half (if you are using a manual system) so they all fit, since you could be eating as many as eight meals in one day.

If you get home in the late afternoon or evening and want to go to a favorite restaurant, this is fine (look at *your* menu choices for this restaurant). You may want to have something ready in your freezer before you leave town, or make a quick trip to the grocery store and pick up a freshly roasted chicken and a side green vegetable, and go home to eat it. Then do your regular grocery shopping the next day if you prefer. Another option is to make breakfast for dinner. Eggs will stay fresh for a week or two, and keep an unopened package of Canadian bacon to use when you return. If you get in late in the evening, depending on your appetite, you may want to just have some cheese and crackers and then go to sleep.

Your meals will be very small and *a little* more lean than usual during this small period of time so that you get back to where you started before you went on vacation. This is only meant for losing weight that you gained from vacation. This routine is not for ongoing weight loss. It won't work, because it will be too restrictive, and your body will not want to eat this way for very long. It is also very time-consuming to eat so often. It is very possible to eat this way and be back to your pre-vacation weight within a few days. If you had vacation constipation, when you get back, everything should start working normally again as well, and will be a significant part of the weight you will lose over the following few days.

The time to get back to your exercise routine is *after* you have had one good night's sleep. *Remember to go back to working out every day.* Based on the kind of vacation you had, follow the guidelines below for getting back into your routine: (Regardless, you should be back to your normal routine within a week.)

» If your vacation was full of activities that kept you moving and physically exerting yourself, then resume your regular exercise routine the day after you come back.

» If your vacation was moderately active (some walking but not physically exerting), cut your routine in half from what you were doing for the first day, and drop your weights by 25 percent, and see how you feel. Progress gradually every day until you are back to your regular routine.
» If your vacation was mostly spent drinking and lying on the beach (good for you!), start out in beginner mode with 15 minute sessions and drop your weights by 50 percent. Increase according to how you feel the next day and the day after.

Airline Travel, et al

There are many ways to travel—by bus, train, ferry, light rail, and commuting. I will be discussing air travel specifically, but the advice can be adapted to all travel when you are away from your ability to eat for more than two hours. You want to be prepared so that you do not make unwise decisions along the way. I am amazed when I look back on my poor decisions for the simplest of things, including picking up a candy bar or eating the free chips or pretzels on a flight. With just a little forethought, I am now able to travel without feeling the negative after affects that used to come with travel. I wouldn't go so far as to say it is just another day, but it is much smoother. When I come home, I rarely find I have put on more than two to three pounds. I take measures to lose it by the end of the first week back—many times it is gone within a couple of days. A lot of this success has to do with the actual travel days themselves.

On the first day of your flight, be sure to eat a good breakfast at home. *You do not need to weigh yourself the day you fly out if you already weighed yourself the morning before.* If your flight is in the morning, feel free to get to the airport early enough to have a good well-balanced breakfast there. There are usually a lot of restaurants past security, but be sure to learn your airport and what each terminal offers so you are not caught off guard with either closed restaurants or only fast food options that may not start your trip off right.

Drink the water you brought with you to the airport until you get to security—flying is dehydrating so you will want to drink a *little* more water that you normally would. Once you are past security, *always*, remember to buy a bottle of water. Be sure you have enough for the time that you will be flying—eight ounces for each hour of flight. You never know when or *if* they will be serving drinks—there could be turbulence during the entire flight.

Pack plenty of nuts and beef jerky for while you are on the plane. Also pack enough for while you are out of town, including late evenings and when you first arrive and everything is closed. Nuts are the easiest food item to port around: mixed nuts, almonds, walnuts, cashews, and pumpkin seeds. You can either get them prepackaged in individual sizes or get a large bag and break them down into small plastic bags.

Personal air travel is a little more relaxed. You do not need to write down what or when you eat or how much you exercise. But that does not mean you do not need to be concerned about such things at all! You don't want to come back from your vacation only to find you have gained more weight than you had allowed for. If you have the opportunity to carry your bags instead of having someone else do it, this will give you some exercise. When you walk through the airport, look for opportunities to keep up the pace and get some great exercise in. Walking while you are on the conveyor belt walkways, and taking the stairs instead of elevators can be great ways to get a little extra exercise in. As always, be safe, and if you have too much luggage, use elevators and/or sky-cabs.

If you fly business or first class, you will probably get a meal on the flight. Make sure that you have not eaten too much within one hour of getting on the plane. Check your flight info to see what is served.

I have been on a three-hour first class flight where all I got were trail mix, pretzels, cookies, and all the booze I wanted—not really the best combination! Check online or call the airline. If you get a meal on your flight, there is usually one meal that is relatively healthy and another that is not so much so. I try to book my seat so that I am in the middle of the pack giving me the best chance of having all options available (they do not have enough of each meal to give to everyone).

It is tempting to eat and drink a lot, since it is all free, but don't do it! You will regret it! Eat normally according to your appetite level at the time. For every three bites of the entrée with protein, I have one bite of the starch and two bites of the vegetable. I rarely eat the dessert that is offered on the flight—it is my own rule. One drink for an hour long flight is more than enough. If the flight exceeds one hour, cut that amount in half per each additional hour and continue to drink water.

Create your rules for whether to eat dessert based on your own desires. I am a chocolate fanatic, so if there is chocolate, I may have a few bites and be fully satisfied. This brings up the touchy issue of wasting food again. There are no leftovers on a plane, so your unconscious or conscious mind may want you to overeat, since it will be otherwise wasted. The saying, "waste here or waist here" is even more important when traveling.

If you are flying coach, be sure you are ready to pay pricey amounts for the more nutritious foods on the flight. The other option is to bring food from home which TSA will allow—be aware of the current rules! (A rule yesterday may not be the same rule today.) There are usually deli's in the airport past security with sandwiches and salads you can bring on your flight...try to think of the possible smell of your foods when deciding what to bring on a plane. Remember that it will be about 1½ hours into your flight before you will be offered any food (assuming there is no turbulence), so be prepared—bring *some* food with you just in case they either run out of what you wanted or are unable to serve the entire cabin.

Things to bring on your carry-on:

- Nuts—unseasoned that you can open and reclose without any fuss or mess
- Cheese sticks—eat within two hours
- Protein bar—well-balanced and not very often
- Trail mix—check to see that it is well-balanced
- Beef jerky
- Water (8 oz. for each hour of flight—per person)

Things to bring in your checked luggage:

- A swimsuit you would swim in (not just to lie on the beach)
- Tennis shoes for walking, running, and working out and comfortable socks
- Comfortable and layered workout clothes (some fitness centers are kept cold)
- Prepackaged easy to eat foods that you can go to instead of the mini-bar
- Flexible bands (and corresponding instructions, if applicable)
- Enough pages of your journal to take you through your trip (for business travel)

Cruise Ships

I was on a cruise, and at the very end, they had a class on how to lose weight while on a cruise ship. I didn't go, but I thought *why wouldn't they have that class at the beginning of the cruise?* Rest assured, you can be on a cruise ship, enjoy everything—including the midnight buffet, and maintain your weight. I know it must seem wasteful to not eat everything that is put in front of you, but I can promise you it is not healthy to eat everything that is put in front of you. All the food on the cruise is free and there will be a lot of waste whether you eat everything you see or not. That is just the way it is. Continually be aware of how your body feels and make sure to not overeat. In fact a cruise is one place where if you feel like eating mini-meals every two hours you can—for free! Although beware of the alcohol bill at the end of the cruise—that is not free!

Driving Trips

You may think that a driving trip would lend itself to eating healthy, since you have so many options available to you, like an ice cooler and the ability to bring foods from home. But more than likely, you have been on a driving trip that went like this:

"I'm hungry!"
"Me, too! What are we going to eat?"
"I don't know—there's a place to eat—let's stop there!"

The next thing you know, you are at a place you have never heard of, and the choices are fried this and fried that, and the best homemade desserts you can imagine. To make it worse, you want to make good time, so you don't want to stop again for another six hours. You overeat so you won't need to stop anywhere except for where? Yep—the gas station!

You can buy healthy foods at the gas station, mini-marts, and almost any restaurant out there, but more than likely, if your trip has already started like this, you aren't going to. Let's start this trip over with a little planning and see how we can make some changes and still allow for some stops along the way if desired.

Before you head out on your trip, decide whether you want to pack all of your food or make a stop or two and eat at a restaurant. If you want to pack all of your food, your best bet is to make sandwiches and cut them in halves or quarters. Be sure your sandwiches are not directly on the ice. There should be a tray above the ice; if not, then put your sandwiches in a hard plastic waterproof container in the ice. If you are eating breadless sandwiches, just pack the sliced meat and cheese, and have them ready to eat. Set your timer on driving trips, since there is a tendency to get bored or restless and want to eat without really addressing whether you are hungry or not. Other people will want to eat on their own time schedules—maintain flexibility without giving up on your goals!

Remember to bring plenty of water, and keep it on ice if you can. Resist the urge to drink soda just because everyone else is doing so. Remember, you are focused on your journey, not theirs! I have a special treat when on a driving trip—an individual bag of Munchos potato chips. I can't seem to find them anywhere except in roadside gas stations. It's my little indulgence that I don't do all the time, and I only go on a couple road trips a year.

Some ideas for sandwiches are:

- Roast beef with cheddar cheese
- Turkey with Swiss cheese
- Ham with provolone
- Pastrami with Havarti cheese

Have some fruit *with* your meals or mini-meals with some dietary fat and protein (not by themselves). Grapes and berries are easy to eat while on the road. For those moments when you just need a snack to make it through to the time that the entire group wants to eat the next meal, have some well-balanced easy options available. Eat just enough to take the edge off your hunger or dizziness. This could be just a quarter of one of the sandwiches. Make sure you do not eat too much—you want to be able to eat with the rest of the group!

Idea's for quick snacks to make it to the next group meal:

» Nuts—almonds, walnuts, or pumpkin seeds
» A quarter of a sandwich
» Cheese slices rolled around celery sticks
» Cheese cubes with a few grapes or berries
» Beef jerky

If you have decided to stop along the way, do not fret. As long as you have decided what town you will stop in ahead of time, you should have an idea of how long before you will eat and be able to gauge when and how much to eat along the way. There is almost always something on the menu that will work with your weight loss journey; you just have to make the decision before you enter the restaurant that you are going to find it! You can even make it into a timing game to see how long it takes you or anyone else who wants to play, to find the best food choice. Avoid the tendency to overeat, because you probably will not be bringing leftovers in the car. Sharing a meal may be the best solution.

Decision Time (to read on now or later)

Now we have gone through everything there is to *losing* weight.

You may want to read the next chapter now, or you may want to wait until you have lost the weight—either is fine. If you decide to read it before you lose the weight, remember that you need to read it again once you do lose the weight. The transition from weight loss to maintaining is critical. There is a lot to it that you do not want to forget once you are at that point in your journey. Read it now and read it again, or wait until you are close or have reached your goal—the choice is yours!

The next and last stop on your weight loss journey is—*Now that You Have Lost the Weight.*

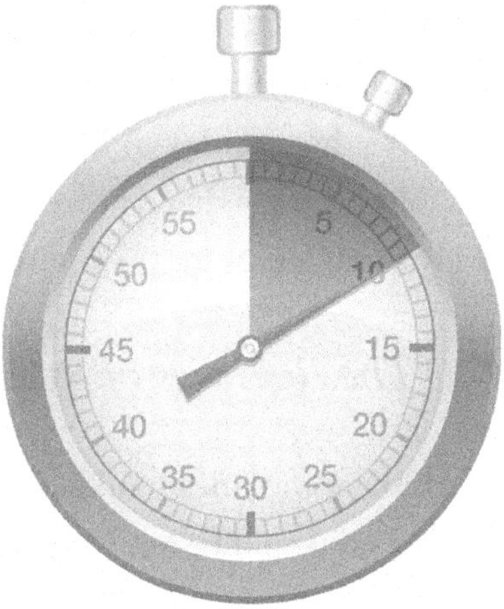

Chapter 9

Now that You Have Lost the Weight

Congratulations!!! I knew you could do it! I really did—you would not have come this far in reading this book and writing in your journals if you weren't committed to reaching your weight loss goals. I am sure you will be surprised by my next piece of advice.

Forget that You Were Ever Overweight!

You may be thinking: *That is absurd, if she thinks I am going to go through all this pain and agony* (well, hopefully not too much pain and agony) *to just forget about it.* But, you want to stay focused on your future and not dwell on the past—not for too long, anyway. Give yourself one month to bask in people's praise. You can tell anyone and everyone (including the checkout clerk when you buy clothes in the size you had only dreamt of months earlier). Bask in this moment; you have earned it! But like with all things that are amazing in life, it is time to move on. Find the next thing to be excited about.

Let's discuss how to know when you are done with your weight loss journey and what do to once you have reached your goals. Are you ready to maintain for the rest of your life and just be you?

The Realities of Reaching Your Weight Loss Goals

I feel like sometimes I am a bubble buster when it comes to what you had hoped would be amazing news (you reached your weight loss goal after all), but the reality may be quite different. The best I can do for you now is to prepare you.

Otherwise, you may be surprised when one-third of the people in your life are very happy for you and think you look amazing, another third think you didn't lose quite enough and you should reconsider your goals, and a surprising final third think you lost too much and went too far in your weight loss journey. So who do you listen to? None of them—you need to listen and look to yourself.

All of these different points of views are just that—other people's views, not yours. How do you know whether there are any valid comments? If the majority of people say you lost too much weight, then you should check in with your doctor and see if the comments are valid. But if the comments are all over the place, then consider yourself lucky. As they say, *you can't please everyone all of the time.*

You need to be happy with yourself. You want to be happy with the size you are in and how you look and feel without clothes as well. Once you exude confidence in your choice of weight, others will begin to see you as you see yourself. Do not let someone's random comment in the future make you doubt your decision.

If you are not prepared, comments or the lack of them can actually cause you to slip up and go backwards and here is the biggest reason why:

> *You will receive so much affirmation for having lost the weight that you may begin to miss all of the attention you were used to getting. Once your significant other, co-worker, and best friend stops telling you how proud they are of you and how awesome you look you may begin to wonder if you still look amazing; trust that you do. But, here's the thing—the other people in your life are already starting to forget that you were overweight, and you need to, also.*

If you do not anchor yourself in feeling confident that you are the right weight for you—right now, before the comments fade away, then you can succumb to the yo-yo dieting that will have you gaining the weight again just so you can feel the affirmation and excitement of losing weight. Working on your new life plans will help you with this transition and provide a new focus.

Another odd phenomenon that can happen once you achieve a goal is the *letdown*. As odd as it may sound, once you get through with the excitement of it all, there can be a feeling of "Is that all there is?"; "Now what?" or "I thought my life would be different!" This is why it really *is* best to forget that you were ever overweight and go forward toward the next chapter in your life. Create new goals and experience new adventures!

How to Know You Are Done with Your Weight Loss Journey

Maybe you are one of those lucky people who picked a goal weight on day one, reached it, are happy with your progress, and are ready to stick to where you are. This is luck, because it does not always go that way. Sometimes you will reach your goal weight and decide you want to go for a little more, and then there is the possibility that you have met your size goal and actually weigh more than you thought. Maybe you just didn't realize how much you would weigh when you were at your goal size. Revising your goals is part of any journey. Take this opportunity to evaluate if you are at the weight you want to stay.

If you decide that you are at the weight you want to be, try it on for size (pun intended) for three months, and make sure you are happy with this new weight and size. Make sure that it is reasonably easy to keep. Sometimes when you lose weight, there is a bounce back of a few pounds, so before you buy a whole bunch of new clothes, sit with your new weight for approximately three months. Then go shopping, and have some fun! You can buy clothes during the three-month time period; just do not buy a lot of expensive clothes until you are committed to your new weight and are sure it suits you!

Plastic Surgery (Should I or Shouldn't I?)

I want to say that I am not a plastic surgery person, but when I reflect on my life and think of the things I have done, I am a little iffy on the subject. I had plastic surgery on my forehead as a child due to two scars I got when I was three and five years old. I am very thankful to my mother for fighting the insurance company to have this plastic surgery when I was young. I also had my veins stripped in the early 90s. I got varicose veins from my pregnancies at a very young age which I guess are hereditary, from my grandma. I tried laser hair removal, but it was not successful for me. I am not against new technology and fixing things to make yourself look better as long as it is safe—however, nothing is ever 100 percent safe; if you do not believe me, read the waiver you will need to sign before you have *anything* done to your body.

The question of surgery needs to be evaluated on a case-by-case situation. I caution that you want to wait until you have finished losing weight with all your own volition. Just remember: If you have any type of surgery related to your looks, you will have to share credit with your surgeon.

Buying New Clothes

Beyond making sure that you are happy with your weight for three months before going crazy with your clothes shopping, make sure that you think about your wardrobe when you go out and buy new clothes. Do you want to change your style or colors that you normally get? Now is the time to do it. I started wearing dresses. I don't remember wearing dresses except for special occasions for years, if not decades! I went out and bought a bikini for the first time in twenty years when I was forty-six. Try some different styles, experiment a little with your new size, and have fun! I put on a pair of designer jeans; they fit really snug (the good kind of snug when you wear jeans with spandex), and someone in the store said they looked amazing! Buying designer jeans was not originally on my to-do list, but I am glad I ventured out and tried them on.

Another thing to keep in mind when buying new clothes is: ***DO get hung up on the size!*** Yes, you heard me right. You worked hard to get into your perfect size; do not let any designer force you to buy a size larger because their sizes run small. This may seem harsh, since you really like a certain pair of jeans, and you know if you just got one more size up, they would look amazing. Besides, the clerk is sure that they run small, so it really isn't like you are buying a larger size. Do not do it! This becomes a slippery slope, and you may find you are not at all bothered by buying the next size up; since you did it once before, you will find it easy to do again. The next thing you know, you are in the larger size and wondering how this happened. Can you buy the next size down due to a designer using vanity sizing? Sure!

I do allow myself to buy one size up in dresses. One caveat—if you do this for a special event, and your weight loss comes up, you will not feel genuine if you say you are one size and are wearing another. If it is a dress for a special occasion, stick to your size, and flaunt it! Do not worry about the size of your swimsuits—buy for the fit, not for the number! Don't forget to check your bra size again and be sure you are wearing the size that flatters your new figure.

Now that you have settled on your size, go ahead and splurge (if you can) so that you have invested in your new weight. Once you have spent a weeks' salary on a new wardrobe and given away all of your bigger clothes (you will soon—when we do the cathartic activity I have been telling you about), you will need to think twice before allowing yourself to gain the weight back again. Don't have a backup plan for *if* you gain the weight back.

What to Do with Your Clothes from Your Past

Now that you have committed to your new weight and are ready to buy new clothes, what do you do with all your old clothes that were a part of your journey? I know it may seem like a good idea to keep them just in case, sell them so you will have more money to buy new clothes, or give them away to charity and get a tax deduction. But, I do not recommend any of these.

If you keep the clothes *just in case*, you are already setting yourself up for *just in case*. When your current jeans start to feel a little tight, you will pull out the *just in case* jeans and run out the door. If you sell your clothes to buy new ones, this will give you positive reinforcement that you can just sell the clothes you are buying right now, and it is no big deal to trade them in, exchange or sell them. If you give your clothes to charity to get the tax deduction, it is the same as selling them; you receive a financial benefit for getting rid of your clothes.

I have a much better idea. I did this with my clothes, and to this day, I still remember the way I felt knowing I was making a difference in someone else's life. I took all the clothes I was ready to give away—dozens and dozens of jeans, suits, dresses, and tops—I boxed them by size, and found someone who needed the specific size that I used to wear. I do not really understand how the Universe works but when I let my request be known that I was looking for people in need, within a week, I heard from three separate people who were in different stages of their lives who really could use the sizes that I had. I either shipped or hand delivered the clothes to each recipient. It was a feel-good moment when I let them go.

> *One person was someone whom I did not know personally but had heard about. The woman recently had bladder surgery. She was required to wear an apparatus inside her clothing, and her current clothes no longer fit. She was a single mom and was not sure how she would be able to afford a new wardrobe for her new medical circumstances. To this day, it makes me grateful that I was able to help someone else through my journey.*

I know some people say to keep your clothes from when you were overweight to remind yourself that you were overweight. But does that make sense for anything else? Do you keep pictures on your desk of your ex-boyfriend so you can remember the past relationship that didn't work out? What if you quit smoking? Do you keep cigarettes around to remind yourself of the bad habit you once had? No, you move on to your future, and you replace your past with your new life. It is important for you to do this now.

Maintaining Your Weight

You may wonder, *isn't there something missing on how I am supposed to keep my weight where it is?* I haven't told you all the secrets yet. If you have ever been able to maintain your weight for three months in your entire life, you have the ability to maintain your weight now without making it a big deal. That's the good news; however, if you have always been all over the place, you will want to pay special attention to the *Rules to Maintain.*

There is not much difference between losing weight and maintaining—and that is on purpose. Whatever you do to lose weight, you must be willing to do to keep it off—almost, anyway. You should have given up one food item that was only for weight loss. Eating the food you gave up during your weight loss journey, will signify that you have met your goals, are happy with your weight, and are ready to live the rest of your life as the new you.

How do you integrate this food back into your life without going crazy? My grandson would make fun of me saying, "I know, Grandma, you only want two french fries." I started out eating only a couple when other people ordered them. I didn't want to go overboard, but I was ready to go forward with my maintenance and the rest of my life, with french fries as a part of it. Now I can enjoy them when the mood strikes, usually with a burger or steak! They actually are a nice reminder of how far I have come and the goals I was able to achieve.

Rules to Maintain

1. ***Continue to eat the way you have been eating.*** Do not eat past the point of feeling just satisfied. You can increase your intake of sugars and starches *just a wee little bit and do so slowly.*
2. ***Weigh yourself every morning.*** Just like you have been doing—it

is very important to do. Keep the same exceptions for vacations, eating holidays, and your birthday.

> *After two years of maintenance and weighing myself every morning, I had new slate flooring put in, making the bathroom floor uneven. I could not get an accurate reading so I put the scale out in my garage. After a couple of months of occasionally remembering to weigh myself (I thought I would know if I were gaining weight), one morning I checked and I was at my YIKES! weight. I immediately found one slate tile in the bathroom that seemed to give me consistent results and I went back to weighing myself every morning!*

3. ***Keep up your daily workout.*** However, if your workouts have been lengthy and you were hoping to reduce them once you met your goals go ahead. Reduce your daily workout by five minutes each day until you are at the daily time you want to be working out.

> *You should aim to workout for about thirty minutes a day as a minimum for the rest of your life! Yes, this may seem like a long time, and hopefully it is. But exercise is known to help the elderly not only with their weight, but also with their memory, bone density, sleep, and overall health. Plan on working out every day—you will not regret it!*

4. ***Keep your weight loss journals from your past.*** These will be the only remnants of your past and are only for reference. Use them to show yourself what you were able to do when things get rough and you doubt your ability to overcome a new obstacle. It can be amazing to scan randomly to see

what you wrote, what you ate, and how much you worked out. I did this when I moved and came across the journals from years ago. It was actually very reaffirming that I had made such a difference in my life and I really was ready for the next journey.

5. ***Continue to write in your journals, as life permits.*** I kept up with my journals daily for a long time after I started maintaining—I skipped a few days here and there. I still find comfort in writing in my journals. If I find myself at my *OMG* weight, I immediately go to my journals to see what I wrote (or did not write).
6. ***Continue to get a good night's sleep.*** Resolve any sleep issues if they persist for more than a few days. Remember you want to feel rested when you wake up!
7. ***Know your comfort weight! Memorize it, and never raise it!*** It is very important to have these numbers in your mind so that you do not find yourself back where you were and wonder how it happened.

Calculating Your Comfort Weight

Your comfort weight is a three-pound range. In this range you know all is well with no worries! First you will need to establish your median weight. During the last three months you have been evaluating whether you are happy with your weight and size. Your median weight is the weight that you have been most often during the last three months. For me, that is 113.0 pounds. My comfort weight is from 112.0 pounds (one pound below my median weight and a weight which I have reached a few times, but not often) all the way up to 114.9 pounds, which is two pounds above my median weight. This is the weight range were I feel comfortable in and out of my clothes and I am most relaxed.

> *When you were losing weight your OMG number was only a one pound range now it is a two pound range. I struggled as to whether I should make them the same, to make it easier to remember. But this is exactly how I did it! The more I looked at why I did it this way, the more it made sense to me. When you are losing weight a three pound fluctuation may not be cause for alarm. While you are maintaining it is important to have an earlier warning signal to begin correction.*

Your *OMG* weight is between two and three pounds above your median weight. So for me my *OMG* weight is 115.0–116.9 pounds and is my notification that I need to make changes to get back to my comfort weight. Your *YIKES!* weight is one pound above your *OMG* weight. For me, 117.0–.9 pounds is a notification that I am in danger and must get back to my comfort weight immediately. Your *never again* weight is five pounds above your median weight. For me, that would be 118.0 pounds or more. You do not want to ever see your *never again* weight!!!

Your *WHOA!* number is a little more than one pound below your median weight. This would be 111.9 for me. Anything close to 112.0 and I know I need to reassess what I am doing so that I do not lose any more weight. This may be a new concept for some people who have always gone as low as they can and see what happens. However, this will cause yo-yo dieting! Do not go lower than your comfort weight. Take steps to *slowly* increase your weight if needed. Eating an entire hot fudge sundae to get back to your comfort weight may seem like a good idea—*it is not!*

What to Do if You End Up at Your OMG or YIKES! Weights

First of all, don't panic! You have what it takes to get yourself back on course. Weighing in at your *OMG* or even your *YIKES!* weight is not a sign of failure. In fact, it is the opposite of failure. You set up your numbers, you weighed yourself every morning, and you noticed immediately there was a problem that needed to be addressed. This is what I call being responsible. You know when to be concerned, and you know (or will know) what to do to fix it!

> *In my line of work, the numbers tell a story, and are provided to the CEO. The CEO looks at them and sees that everything is okay or that some issues need to be addressed right away. This is responsible. The CEO who doesn't analyze the numbers—or worse, doesn't even ask for the numbers to be calculated until it is too late—may find that the company has too big of a problem and may not be able to recover. Do not let this happen to you!*

How to get back to your comfort weight as soon as possible:

» Get a good night's sleep (8–9 hours)

» If you haven't been writing in your journals, go back to writing in them now

» Decrease the amount that you eat at each meal so you are just *barely* satisfied—that point is a *little* before you are completely satisfied

» Increase the intervals between meals so that you eat every 2–3 hours

- Be sure to include dietary fat, protein, and carbohydrates with every meal
- If you have been skipping your workouts, get out and walk, or do something for 30 minutes a day—not necessarily all at once
- If you normally drink alcohol daily (I am not saying that you should, but if you do), only have one drink per day until you are back to your comfort weight

What to Do When You Lose Weight Unexpectedly

There may be times in your life once you have reached what you thought was your perfect weight that you lose weight unexpectedly. Sickness, tragedy, a breakup, and bouts of stress can all cause your weight to plummet suddenly and unexpectantly, and you may be too preoccupied with the current situation to deal with the weight loss. You need to wait it out and see if this is temporary or permanent.

> *I did not want to lose weight. I was very happy at a size 4; it was my ideal weight while I wrote the majority of this book. I actually was alarmed when I lost the weight so suddenly. My jeans were hanging off of me after an hour of wearing them. I was sad about having lost my daughter, so I was crying daily, and the last thing I wanted to worry about was my weight. I know I ate throughout the days; I really just assumed it would come back eventually once I was able to calm myself down, even though I wasn't sure how that was possible.*
>
> *After five months, I realized that my body had just adapted to the weight loss, and it was what it was. Very reluctantly, I went ahead and purchased clothes in size 2 and decided to*

> *keep my size 4 clothes for a year, just in case. I decided this was okay, since size 4 was my goal, I had no desire to be a size 2, and I had been size 4 for almost three years. So far, I have stayed a size 2 for over a year now and have grown to accept and reluctantly embrace it. But I would have been fine if I had gone back to a size 4. I have not given away my size 4s yet; not because I want them just in case, but because I know what they mean and I am not quite ready to say good-bye.*

If you lose weight unexpectedly after you have reached your goal and purchased your wardrobe, wait at least three months before going out and buying a new wardrobe. Then put the entire old wardrobe away for one year—just to be sure you are settled into the new weight and size. Then give away the clothes in the way that feels best to you.

What to Do Once You Lose the Weight

Well, that is the question isn't it? I feel a certain freedom by not having to worry about my weight. I have my *OMG* days, and on a very rare occasion a *YIKES!* day; but I have not had a *never again* day. I know what it takes to make my weight a non-issue and keep my comfort weight. I have problems just like everyone does, but I can mark weight loss off the list—no more New Year's resolutions to lose 10 pounds or workout more often—since you only make goals for things you are not doing.

Rest assured I have plenty of areas in my life that I want to make improvements in, and now I have the time to devote to them. I have the confidence that has carried forward from being able to lose weight without sacrificing my own needs and by creating my own rules. I want you to go forward and use this feeling of accomplishment toward your next journey! So join me and raise your glass, congratulate yourself, and make your next goal!

With all my love and admiration for the path you have chosen,
Sherri Sue Fisher

Appendix A

Grocery Lists

Your first line of defense in making good food choices is at the grocery store!

Let's face it if you don't buy it, you can't eat it. This is where your home situation can be an issue. Let's assume that you have some significant control over what your kids eat, they may complain at first, but most likely, you will be able to get them to eat a wide variety of foods that are also good for them *and* will be good for you as well. Desserts are not necessarily off-limits; you just want to have some effort exerted in order to have them available. Learning the basics of cooking is great for all kids, so have them do age-appropriate things in the kitchen with you and learn in the process.

What about the other adults in the house for which you really do not have much control? This is where you need to tread cautiously. Is something that others truly want one of your trigger foods? You can always ask if they wouldn't mind if this particular trigger food wasn't in the house for a while—at least until you felt you had more control over your impulses. If they say no, this food or drink is really important to them, or you decide not to even ask, then you will need to desensitize yourself to this particular food or drink. I did this with soda. I trained myself to think of soda as only something I drank when I was sick. I keep ginger ale in my refrigerator at all times, and I have no desire to drink it unless my stomach is upset.

It's kind of a mind game, but you say to yourself what you want to feel about a certain food or drink whenever you see it. If potato chips are in the house because the other adult wants to continue eating them, you could say to yourself, "Not in my best interest," "Those will make me sick," or "I'd rather eat something more substantial." Once you find a saying that resonates with you, then continue that same saying every time you see what you want to avoid. The saying can be different for different things. You can have one saying for potato chips and another for soda, like "Only when I am sick!" After a while, you will notice that you automatically say this message to yourself whenever you see this particular item.

Creating Grocery Lists by Categories

Below are *ideas* for your grocery shopping list by categories. This list is not meant for you to go to the store and buy everything on it. You will want to create your own list, whether it is on paper, on the computer, or using an app. Categories will make grocery shopping faster and less likely to buy something you do not need. Also, there is less possibility of forgetting something because you have to go to the other side of the store since you didn't notice it on your list the first time. Have your menus already figured out so you buy foods that go together and therefore, less chance of spoiling.

Dairy Case

There are so many different kinds of cheeses to choose from, try experimenting but be sure to check the price so you do not get sticker shock at the checkout counter. Most of the cheeses here are low to moderately priced. But, some cheeses can be very expensive. Do not buy reduced-fat, low-fat, or fat-free options of anything!

» Eggs—enough for at least one per day
» Hard-boiled eggs—prepackaged and already peeled
» Cottage cheese (4 percent fat)
» Butter (Grade A or better)
» Half and half for coffee (real only)
» Whole milk (if you are a milk drinker)
» Cheddar cheese of any kind (a block that you slice yourself for night time)
» Thinly sliced cheese for sandwiches or breadless sandwiches
» Cheese sticks or squares (1 oz. individually pre-wrapped) to take on the run
» Mozzarella cheese (the kind that is in a ball)
» Goat cheese (creamy kind to put on crackers—plain or herb and garlic are good)
» Shredded and/or grated parmesan cheese
» Feta or blue cheese crumbles (for salad)

Fresh Fruits and Vegetables

There are many options, so I will just point out my favorites, and you can add or delete from there. I only buy a few fruits and vegetables each week and try to change what I get as the seasons and sales allow. I also get enough salad fixings to have several during the week. I get the smallest batch of bananas I can find and keep a few on hand all the time.

Fruits

- Bananas
- Strawberries
- Pears
- Peaches
- Plums
- Apples
- Oranges
- Blueberries
- Blackberries
- Raspberries
- Cherries
- Grapes
- Watermelon
- Pineapple

Vegetables

- Broccoli
- Zucchini
- Squash
- Potatoes
- Asparagus
- Corn on the cob
- Green beans
- Spinach
- Cauliflower
- Carrots
- Mushrooms
- Green Beans
- Peas
- Salsa (deli premade or the makings)

Salad Fixings

- Red onions
- Romaine heart or any lettuce

- On-the-vine tomatoes
- Roma tomatoes
- Artichoke hearts (jarred marinated in seasonings)
- Green onions (scallions)

Canned and/or Frozen Vegetables vs. Fresh—Cooked, or Raw

You should keep some canned and/or frozen vegetables on hand for those times when the fresh ones have gone bad, you are ready to make a meal, and there is no time or desire to go to the grocery store. It happens to the best of us, and there is nothing wrong with including canned and frozen vegetables in your menu plan when fresh foods are not available. Always check your expiration dates before opening a can or using your frozen foods.

Also, some vegetables taste very different fresh-cooked instead of raw and frozen instead of canned. Your preferences can be from the way you were brought up. One specific vegetable that comes to mind is cauliflower, I love it raw, but I do not care for it cooked. While spinach I love canned and I don't feel that I do it justice when I try to cook it myself. If you have never eaten a vegetable a certain way, venture out, and if you aren't used to cooking fresh vegetables—check out *Appendix B—Cooking* for some easy ways to add fresh cooked vegetables to your meals!

Deli Meats

I almost always go to the deli counter (unless it is closed) and get the best brand of deli meats the store has. If you want to get nitrate-free, there are brands of deli-meat that do not contain nitrates; be sure to ask if this is a concern. If you do not already have your favorites, ask for a taste. You do not need a lot to make sure that you like it. You also do not want to buy something only to find out it does not taste the way you thought it would. If the meat is precut and doesn't look very fresh or isn't the thickness that you want, do not hesitate to ask for your deli meat to be sliced fresh. There is no need to buy a full pound if you do not want to; you can order as small as a 1/8 lb. if that is all you need. They will usually only stay fresh for a few days.

My favorite deli meats are:

- Roast beef
- Pepper turkey
- BBQ chicken
- Pastrami
- Honey Ham

Fish, Steak, and Chicken

Keep enough fish, steak, and/or chicken in the freezer to make a meal for when you do not have time to go grocery shopping. Remember to use what you have frozen and rotate out based on the guidelines for freezing times in your all-purpose cookbook. Look at *Appendix B—Cooking* for information on how to thaw quickly and safely. Most chicken and fish entrées can be baked, making for easy to prepare meals.

Here are my favorites:

- Fish—frozen with or without toppings (not breaded)
- Halibut
- Mahi Mahi
- Tilapia
- Grouper
- Swordfish
- Sea Bass
- Fish—fresh (should be eaten the day purchased)
- Salmon

- Shrimp (so easy and very fast in a skillet)
- Crab
- Steak—any kind that you like and feel is priced well (try to have at least four days left on the expiration date—unless you plan to eat it sooner)
- Shredded or ground beef—quality beef is important; ask your butcher
- Chicken—organic is best
- Breasts are good for grilling
- Tenders are good for fajitas (skip the tortillas and add lots of veggies)

Beverages

This is definitely a personal preference—but my recommendation is to minimize the alcohol consumption while losing weight except for special occasions or social events. There were many days that I did not drink alcohol, and did not miss it, and then there were days where I did drink alcohol and still lost weight the next morning. I don't really know the answer, except to keep track of what you do and see if you notice a pattern.

- Champagne or sparkling wine—seems to not affect weight loss like wine, beer, and mixed drinks can
- Coffee (flavored is fine—no syrups)
- Tea (any kind)
- Water—you may decide to buy or not buy (some people prefer their local water)

Grains

You will eat *some* grains daily. Choose wisely so that you are able to enjoy without guilt. You want to think about the size of your breads along with the freshness. If you have a bakery onsite at your grocery store, see what they have to offer. Avoid oversized breads unless you are able to eat only a half a slice. Sourdough is an example of bread that can be very large and may need to be cut in half. If you like whole wheat then buy it, if you like rye bread—then go for it! You should enjoy the grains you eat. I do not care for whole wheat, but I do enjoy multi-grain once in a while. English muffin toasting bread and sourdough are my favorites. This was something I did not like on many diets and is not a restriction on the *Timer DIET* program. If you like white bread I see no problem eating white bread, if you can get your bread from the bakery that would be ideal.

Pasta is a grain that you will want to eat in small quantities especially if you are in weight loss mode. A little pasta can go a long way in meeting your carbohydrate intake—there are protein-enriched pastas now that I have found to be delicious, you may want to consider them when choosing your pastas.

My favorite grains are:

- Saltine crackers
- Bread (fresh from the bakery—English muffin toasting bread)
- Pasta (protein-enriched pasta)

Desserts

Ideally, desserts should be made from scratch or from fruits, perhaps adding some heavy cream or making it into whipped cream. Avoid the temptation to buy premade desserts from the grocery store—they will be too easy to get to. There are a few exceptions of desserts to have on hand if you feel you need to.

Premade desserts

- Chocolate squares (at least 60 percent dark cacao) are great to keep on hand. One to three of these squares are very satisfying. Eat them slowly, and savor every bite.
- Natural vanilla or chocolate ice cream (no extra candies—no fat-free either)
- Angel food cake (from the bakery is okay) to add fresh strawberries to

Homemade desserts

- Ice cream—either with or without an ice cream maker
- Homemade brownies (with flour, sugar, and eggs!)
- Fresh fruit (with or without freshly made whip cream)

Spices vs. Sauces

If you use spices rather than sauces, you will minimize unneeded sugars. I love teriyaki sauce, but add it to pork tenderloin, and you increase the carbohydrates by up to five grams. Instead, you could add almost any seasoning, and there would be no sugar, thus no carbs and no extra calories! That is not to say you can *never* have sauce; just remember that it may be *not in your best interest* while you are on your weight loss journey. Instead, try these spices to enhance the flavor of all your foods, including your vegetables:

- Kosher salt or sea salt—large chunks
- Garlic salt
- Seasoned salt
- Black pepper kernels (freshly ground)
- Italian seasonings
- Mexican seasonings

- » Cinnamon chips with grinder (on toast and fruit is great!)
- » Raw sugar
- » Almost any type of spices that you like!

Don't be afraid to ask friends and your favorite restaurant about a certain spice you like. Most will be happy to tell you (even if they won't give you the recipe!).

Salad and Salad Dressings

Put your salad in a watertight container and shake the salad. You will use less dressing, and it will get all over the salad and not be concentrated in one area. Your salads do not need to be anything fancy—lettuce, tomatoes, and an onion is great. Add some chopped walnuts or sliced almonds for some crunch.

Salad dressings that are fresh and do not have preservatives in them are best. The fewer preservatives in your life, the better; I don't think anyone can argue with that. You can't get rid of processed foods and preservatives entirely without a *lot* of effort and commitment. You don't really have to have them completely out of your life, but you do need to make a concerted effort to eliminate them whenever given the opportunity.

Frozen Dinners and Combination Foods

You may wonder why I have these in the same area. Their labels can be misleading—in a good way. Sometimes complete meals or foods that require assembly will base food values on you eating the entire contents. If you are able to take out the portions that you know are *not in your best interest*, like croutons, sauce with sugar in it, or some pasta or dressing, you can make these meals much more doable and within reason—more well-balanced. Look at the package, and see if there is something that you can eliminate to make it good option. They are great to have on hand when you do not have time to cook.

What's in My Fridge?

I woke up one morning while in the middle of writing my book and decided I should write down what is in my refrigerator and so here it is:

Strawberries
Raspberries
Pineapple
Watermelon
Bananas (not in refrigerator)
Red onion
Half-and-half quart
Cottage cheese (4% fat)
Hummus Three-Pepper
Shredded parmesan cheese
Blue cheese wedge
Shredded sharp cheddar cheese
Sharp cheddar cheese block
Cheddar cheese sticks and squares
Hard-boiled eggs (peeled)
Dozen eggs
Sourdough bread (bakery)
Caesar salad dressing
Honey Dijon dressing
Sparkling wine
Butter
Neufchâtel cheese
Goat cheese
Bacon
Deli roast beef
Smoked salmon (for salads)
Tomatoes on the vine
Pre-sliced white mushrooms
Baby carrots in a bag
Broccoli (fresh)
White potato
Sweet potato
Garlic clove
Mayonnaise
Green olives stuffed with garlic
Sour cream
Salsa (fresh, medium spice)
Leftovers (steak and beans)
Pumpkin spice spread (impulse buy)
Red raspberry pomegranate juice
Real lemon juice
Ginger ale (only if I am sick!)

Margarita in a bottle (two years old!)
Dill pickles
Grated canned parmesan cheese
Vitamin water *(6 mos. old—for hangover)*
Bailey's
Deli Swiss cheese slices
Fiji water
Ice wine
Lemon liqueur

I hope this gives you an idea of how everyday foods can make for a rational way to lose weight and be enjoyable at the same time!

Appendix B

Cooking

The less glamorous side of cooking is dirty dishes—and worse, a dirty kitchen! My grandma taught me to clean as you go, and that lesson has served me well, especially when it comes to baking, large family dinners, and romantic dinners for two. When it comes to the end of the meal, I am pretty much ready to run the dishwasher, and everything is put away. Some things that belong in the refrigerator will be easier to remember since you will want to put them away immediately so they stay fresh. There are other things that might not be so obvious: Keep your dishwasher ready for dirty dishes so that when you are done making something in the kitchen, it can go straight into the dishwasher.

My normal routine is to run the dishwasher every night so that in the morning, while I make breakfast, I can unload the dishwasher and be ready for the dishes from breakfast and the rest of the day. You may need to run your dishwasher more often; it can make the difference between dreading cooking vs. enjoying it.

Not having a system figured out can also mess with your plans if the dishes you need are dirty or if you really want to clean up and the dishwasher is already full. Also, if you use something that cannot be put into the dishwasher, you will have to wash it by hand—this may not make you very happy. You may want to make changes to what you have in your kitchen if what you need to use often is not dishwasher safe or does not fit into your dishwasher.

Always keep your counters clean! I love paper towels, but my grandmother would have said that is a waste of money and that I should always use real towels and wash them frequently. Whatever you choose, keep your counters clean, especially when dealing with foods like raw eggs and chicken, as there can be bacteria transferred onto other foods. Wash your hands with an unscented soap before you begin cooking—you do not want your food tasting like lavender. If you must—use vanilla or lemon scent; however, if you aren't working with something like chicken or raw eggs, you can just rinse off your hands without soap while in the middle of your cooking.

As you get to know how to cook better, you will find that you can make up your own recipes. Be sure to write them down while you make them. I cannot tell you how many times I have made something only to have everyone love it and ask me how I made it, and I have no idea! I started using my journals to write down the ingredients when I was creating a new recipe and if it turned out amazing, then I wrote it in a more permanent place and saved it for another time.

You can also swap or omit items when you are cooking; it is not like baking. Baking requires exactness in amounts, brands, and ingredients. If your recipe calls for flour, baking soda, or baking powder—then follow the recipe exactly. But when cooking, you can usually experiment with everything except temperatures—make sure your food is cooked thoroughly, by adhering to the exact temperature and cooking time. But, if the recipe calls for bell pepper and you are not a fan, swap them out for something like a red onion, or just omit them altogether.

Cooking Vegetables

Cooking vegetables can be intimidating if you are only used to opening a can or making a salad—at least it was for me. I learned the ease of steaming, the art of grilling, and the thrill of sautéing in very little time. Below are various ways to cook vegetables that will enhance any entrée you make.

Steamed: Put water into the bottom pot of the steamer so that there is an inch or two between the water and the bottom of the basket of the steamer that will be put on top of the bottom pot—do not put the vegetables in the steamer until the water is boiling—they can be left alone—but do not forget about them, set a timer to remind yourself they are on the stove. Cooking time depends on the vegetable, carrots and corn on the cob will take substantially longer than broccoli or asparagus. You can put a fork in the vegetable to see if it is tender and ready to remove from the steamer.

Great vegetables for the steamer:

- Broccoli
- Carrots

- Cauliflower
- Asparagus
- Green beans
- Corn on the cob (may require some turning over)

Grilled: Marinate with an oil based salad dressing or put butter on your vegetables before putting them on the grill; this will keep them from drying out. Aluminum foil is a great barrier between your vegetables and the flame from the grill. Always make sure the pieces are large enough that they do not fall into the grill. Using shish kabobs or a pan that is made for the grill are also good alternatives.

Popular grilled vegetables:

- Baked potato
- Corn on the cob
- Asparagus
- Onions
- Mushrooms

Sautéed: Thinly slice your vegetables first and then put either butter or olive oil in the pan and heat at medium to medium-high—stir often with a spatula until lightly brown—do not leave them for even a few seconds.

Easy to sauté vegetables:

- Zucchini
- Squash
- Mushrooms
- Onions
- Green Onions (scallions)
- Potatoes

Basic Terms of Cooking

If you are not familiar with cooking terms you will want to learn the following basic cooking terms:

- **Fold:** A gentle "folding" motion with a spatula (like you would a sweater)
- **Stir:** A circular motion not too fast, not gentle either using a spoon
- **Pinch:** The spice you are "pinching" is usually in a cup and you "pinch" it like you would a cheek this is the amount they are referring to—it is smaller than a **dash** which is about two pinches.
- **Sauté:** A small amount of fat (butter/oil) in a pan on the stove at medium to med-high, so as to lightly brown
- **Simmer:** Simmering can be done from the beginning starting out on a low heat or it can be done after something has come to a boil and then you bring it back down to a "simmer" lowering the temperature immediately after it has reached the boiling point. Simmering will produce *little* bursts of bubbles when reached.
- **Cut:** This is a very basic term and could mean *anything.* You can either "cut" the way you would like or select a specific cutting technique, such as dicing, chop, or Julienne strips—there are many ways to cut including in half.
- **Chop:** The main focus of chop is the size—each piece should be small, no bigger than a half-inch diameter. Chop is not intended to produce uniform pieces of food, so feel free to *chop* away.

Cooking Tips

Thawing meats and fish is very easy. Fill up your sink or a bowl with cool tap water. If your tap water is on the warm side, then add a few ice cubes (before putting your frozen food in the water); you want your water to be slightly cool and deep enough that the entire frozen item will be covered in the cool water. Keep the frozen item in the plastic bag that it was frozen in, and immerse it in the water. It will float to the top; put something heavy on top of it so that the frozen item stays entirely immersed in the water. Make sure that whatever you put on top of the frozen item to keep it in the water does not fall off, thus causing it to float again. When thawing more than one package, be sure they are not touching each other.

Check the item after 15 minutes. It may already be thawed; if not, then begin checking every five minutes. You should be able to squish the middle without feeling anything frozen. Do not let it thaw longer than absolutely needed; it will get warm fast and may spoil. I do not recommend thawing your food in the refrigerator, since this method can take hours—it may not be thawed when you are ready to cook or your plans for dinner may have already changed. Do not mix methods for thawing!

Microwaving is great for reheating. But unless your particular meal was specifically designed for the microwave, (e.g., TV dinners) do not use the microwave for cooking. I definitely use the microwave for reheating—I know how easy it is to ruin a great leftover meal in seconds. Start slowly; five seconds can mean the difference between a warm medium-rare steak and a well-done steak. Reheat foods once and only once. Take out only what you feel you will eat and place in a microwavable safe dish or plate, and put the rest back in the refrigerator. Throw away what you have reheated and did not eat.

My friend taught me the 70/30 rule when I complained about how much effort it took to grill. I found out, when grilling, you only flip once! When you first put your meat on the grill, keep it there for

70 percent of the total time, and when you flip, only 30 percent of the total time is left. Then wrap your meat in aluminum foil for five minutes, and your meat will be nice and juicy! (This works for chicken breasts and certain fish that is thick like swordfish.) There are too many variations to provide exact grilling times and temperature. Check your general all-purpose cookbook for the food you want to grill and what temperature you desire for estimated grilling times.

Baking an entrée is a favorite of mine, since it is so easy! Chicken and fish are the easiest to bake. If you buy something that has baking instructions, then follow them exactly. If not, you can use a cookbook to get estimates of the time and temperature to set your oven to. There are also thermometers that you can insert into your food that will let you know when the desired temperature is achieved. I use aluminum foil on my broiler pans for easy clean up. I sometimes second-guess myself, so I cut into the middle to make sure it is thoroughly cooked. (Great cooks do not need to do this, but I do not consider myself a great cook yet.)

Timing will come more naturally to others. If you are having difficulty with everything being ready at the same time, take a few minutes and write down how long each item should take you then write down the exact time you will need to start each item so that they are ready at the same time. After a while this part of the process will become much easier.

Cooking is about trial and error and not giving up! Keep it simple, and continue to try new foods in and out of the home. Some of my best ideas have come from trying to duplicate what I had at a restaurant. If you really feel you need a cooking class, go for it—but you probably don't.

Appendix C

Menus and Restaurant Guide

This section will be your go to section for getting started, while you are on your journey, and even when you are in maintenance mode. Everything begins with the menus and what *you* decide to eat.

Menus

Break your menus into various segments so you will be able to select from the one that fits your current situation. There may be some duplication; if so, that's fine. You want to have a separate menu for breakfast, one menu for lunch/dinner, and another for mini-meals. Lunch and dinner are very similar, so I do not differentiate. That is not to say that if you want breakfast for dinner, you could not just look to your breakfast menu and decide on an omelet at dinnertime. Further breakdown your menus by how long they take to make. When you are selecting a menu also think about how long it will take to eat (if time is a factor). Salads actually take a long time to eat, so if I am in a hurry, I would not pick a salad; I would pick a sandwich or something on a cracker that will satisfy me in less amount of time.

Choosing Foods to Include in Your Menus

Your menus must be made before you start your weight loss journey—when you are hungry is no time to decide what would make good combinations of food. Each meal or mini-meal needs to have dietary fat, protein, and carbohydrates of similar proportions. You do not need a calculator or anything fancy—just basic fundamentals of what each type of food has.

You may be tempted to cut down on or cut out the dietary fat in an attempt to lose weight fast, but it won't work—and if it does, it will be at a high cost to your body and overall health. Dietary fat does not make you fat; overeating gives you excess weight. Stick with the principles of making sure that all three are present in your meals or mini-meals, and you will see gradual weight loss.

Make a list of all the foods that you like, love, *and* hate. Why do I include *hate*? You need to assess these foods carefully. Do you really hate them? Is it possible you had a bad experience or maybe you "think" you hate it and haven't tried it or it has been decades? Maybe you liked it at a restaurant but would not dare to try to make it at home? What about foods you have never tried—I can't believe I didn't have a bagel until I was in my early 20s. I also didn't have guacamole until my 30s. Some people have never had rhubarb pie or fried okra; I had both when

I was a child, so did my kids and they loved the fried okra. Take this time to reevaluate your likes and dislikes and see if they are still valid.

Write down any foods or drinks that you love and are not sure you are allowed to have. Then ask yourself these questions:

» Why do I think I am not allowed to eat this food? Or, drink this drink?
» Does this food cause me to eat in excess? Is it a possible trigger food?
» Can I have this food once in a while? Or, is it a food I eat all the time?
» Is this something I really should give up, because it is *not in my best interest*?
» Is there something else I can have instead that would make me just as satisfied?

These are questions you need to answer for yourself. Answer as honestly as you can, and then decide what is best for you!

You want to know what groceries to buy—and that all starts with your menus. It is important to not go overboard and buy *all* the groceries for *all* of your menu ideas; that would cost a lot of money! Try to stick to a few fruits and vegetables each time you shop, and switch them up for variety. When creating your menus, try to do what my grandma always said, "Have at least one green vegetable at lunch and at dinner." Choose one that you already feel comfortable working with. Familiarity will help give you momentum. The simplest way to prepare most vegetables is either raw or to steam them and add just a little melted butter, seasoning, or salt and pepper. Check out *Appendix B—Cooking*, especially if this is all new to you or would like a refresher course on the basics of the kitchen.

Be sure to have different textures in your menu options. Some crunch is needed several times a day. You don't have to have crunch at every meal, but at least a few of your meals should have some type of crunch to them. Toast counts as crunch. I toast my bread for my sandwiches. Crackers are also a great way to add crunch to your meals. Your mind and body want variety, so it is important to have a variety of temperatures and textures woven into your menus.

For foods you routinely incorporate into your meals, knowing what the *approximate* ratios based on grams of dietary fat, protein, and carbohydrates are will make mealtime easier. Here are some of the foods I routinely eat, that I keep memorized:

» Cheddar cheese: 60% dietary fat and 40% protein
» Eggs: 40% dietary fat and 60% protein
» Canadian bacon: 2% dietary fat and 98% protein
» Steak tenderloin: 30% dietary fat and 70% protein
» Chicken breasts: 10% dietary fat and 90% protein
» Tuna fish: 1% dietary fat and 99% protein
» Vegetables: Mostly carbohydrates. However, some have significant sources of protein and/or dietary fat—so if you need more specific information check each vegetable
» Fruit: Mostly carbohydrates
» Cottage cheese with 4%-milkfat: 20% dietary fat, 60% protein, and 20% carbohydrates
» Fried anything: Mostly fat for the fried portion
» Saltine crackers: 1% dietary fat, 1% protein, and 98% carbohydrates
» Pasta—protein enriched: 15% protein and 85% carbohydrates
» English muffin toasting bread: 5% dietary fat, 20% protein, and 75% carbohydrates

When deciding on your meals for the week, remember that your fresh fish must be eaten first, your poultry second, and your beef third; freeze all foods that you have not eaten by their due date or the day before if you already know you won't prepare them the next night.

You cannot refreeze anything! Do not thaw foods until you are ready to cook them. It only takes 15–30 minutes to defrost almost anything; check out *Appendix B—Cooking* for instructions on how to do this.

Creating Your Menus

The menus below are just ideas; feel free to use them, add to them, or delete them from *your* menus. As always, eat only until the point of feeling satisfied and be sure to eat some of everything so you maintain a well-balanced meal. In other words, do not eat all of your toast with butter and only a bite or two of your egg—you want to maintain balance in what you eat as well, even if you do not eat all of your meal.

Breakfast (Less than Five Minutes to Make)

- Hard-boiled egg with a small tomato and green onion; add a little kosher or sea salt
- Mock banana split: ½ cup 4% fat cottage cheese, 1 sliced strawberry, ¼ banana (sliced), and 2 small chunks pineapple, cut into bite size pieces
- Egg(s) scrambled, over easy, fried or sunny-side-up with either ham, bacon, Canadian bacon, chorizo, add a small piece of fruit and one slice of toast with melted butter
- Omelet—add anything that sounds good, try adding different spices and salsa for ways to change it up—don't forget to add shredded cheese

Breakfast (Five to Fifteen Minutes to Make)

» Poached egg on top of half of an English muffin with butter without the hollandaise sauce
» Eggs anyway you like them, with a piece of meat and a pancake (also a great dinner!)
» Frittata with eggs, ham, green onions, and cheese

Leftovers for Breakfast (With Additional Cooking)

» Leftover spinach or crabmeat included in your omelet for breakfast
» Leftover enchiladas add an egg (over easy) on top
» Leftover Steak and eggs with a small piece of fruit

Mini-Meals (Less than Five Minutes to Make)

» Crackers with peanut butter and mashed fruit (bananas and berries are good)
» Hard-boiled egg with tomatoes and kosher salt
» Goat cheese spread *thickly* on crackers
» Blue cheese and watermelon
» Prosciutto and cantaloupe
» Crackers with deli pepper turkey
» Cheddar cheese with fresh fruit
» Cottage cheese with fruit

Easy Lunches and Dinners (Less than 10 Minutes to Prepare)

» Pepper turkey on saltine crackers with a side dish of tomatoes, kosher salt, and pepper
» Tuna with hard-boiled egg, mayo, salt, and pepper (you may want to put in refrigerator about an hour ahead of time to allow

the seasonings to marinate a little). Then put the tuna salad on saltine crackers or on a bed of lettuce add tomatoes

- Roast beef on toasted bread with mayo and sliced red onions
- Mozzarella and tomatoes with salt and pepper and balsamic vinegar
- Grilled cheese sandwich and a small cup of tomato soup (no crackers)
- Roast beef, cherries, cheddar cheese, and hard-boiled egg
- Club sandwich—deli turkey, bacon, tomatoes, lettuce, and cheese on toast with mayo
- Bacon, lettuce, and tomato (with or without cheese) sandwich
- Chicken precooked on a bed of lettuce with shredded cheese and red onions—dressing is half salsa and half ranch dressing

Sandwiches: Start with only half a sandwich. That is usually enough. Toast your bread if you want some crunch. Stack your sandwich so half is more than enough—double the goodies and half the bread! It is better to eat a quarter of a sandwich that is full of goodies than a whole sandwich that has barely anything in it!

Leftovers (Less than One Minute—in most cases)

You should eat all of your leftovers! This way of thinking and acting will allow you to *not* overeat, because you will know that you really will eat your leftovers before they spoil. Most leftovers are good for another day or two after you come home. Be sure to bring them straight home and do not leave them in the car. I have heard people say, "Oh, I never eat my leftovers, so I really don't want to waste my food!" What a waste to your waist!

If you have enough leftovers for more than one meal, only reheat the amount for this meal, and keep the rest in the refrigerator for the next meal or mini-meal.

Baked vs. Grilled Lunches or Dinners

The only difference is that with the grilled food, you will need to flip once, and with the baked food, you shouldn't need to flip at all. A side benefit is that you can workout while your lunch or dinner is cooking! Or you can play with the kids or read a book—you do not need to stand over the food as it cooks! Just set your timer close to you so you do not forget about your meal! Some ideas to get you started:

Baked Choices

» Tilapia, salsa, and cheddar cheese
» Tilapia, tomato sauce, and parmesan cheese
» Chicken—stuffed with spinach and mozzarella cheese with Italian seasonings
» Cornish game hen
» Lasagna

Grilled Choices

» Salmon with seasonings
» Swordfish with drawn butter
» Steak and baked potato with butter and cheese

Dinner with or without Microwave (Less than 10 Minutes)

» Pork tenderloin (precooked)—microwave in thirty-second increments for up to five minutes, opening the microwave door in between each thirty-second increment to avoid over-cooking.

Cover lightly with a paper towel to avoid splattering. Canned yams cook on the stovetop at medium heat for three minutes.

- Chili with beans, shredded cheddar cheese, and sliced onions—cook on the stovetop on medium heat for three to five minutes.
- Frozen fish that is prepackaged with a chimichurri sauce—microwave per the instructions—it should be about ten minutes. Also, some frozen fish have instructions to go straight to the oven and will be ready in less than 30 minutes. Asparagus and broccoli are vegetables that can be steamed in just a few minutes.
- Salad as an entrée—romaine lettuce (or whatever lettuce you like), red onion slices, tomatoes, other veggies that you like and add some protein:
- leftover chicken, steak, or salmon heated slightly in microwave for five to ten seconds or sliced cold and added to salad
- grilled chicken strips—precooked from the deli or meat department
- smoked salmon—thick, meaty cold precooked
- hard-boiled egg—sliced or diced
- chopped walnuts or sliced almond

Light Dinner or a Late Night Mini-meal

- Goat cheese and crackers
- Fruit and semi-hard cheese
- Cottage cheese and fruit
- Caprese salad
- Hard-boiled egg and tomato
- Braunschweiger on crackers
- Deli ham or turkey slices on crackers

Restaurant Guide

It is just as important to have menus already figured out for when you are not at home and need to make decisions that will affect your weight loss goals. Knowing your options ahead of time and having them somewhere easily accessible will make this easier for you. Here are some ideas:

Fast Food Items

- Taco—hard shell with beef, with or without sour cream
- Egg sandwich (no croissants)
- Cheeseburger (no fries and eat half of the bun—using either the fake bun technique or by cutting in half or skip the bun altogether and have a few fries)
- Chicken nuggets or chicken tenders (*no* sauce—you may be surprised how good they really taste without the sugary sauce)

Vending machines are a little tricky, since you are not able to see the nutritional content until you buy it—yet! Let's go over your best bets:

- Nuts—peanuts are good, mixed nuts are great, trail mix is a mixed bag (pun intended)—do not eat a lot of the raisins, very little of the cracker sticks, and none of the dried fruit, which is nothing but sugar!
- Beef jerky is a safe bet, especially if it is the real kind; the sticks are fine and sometimes come in a package with cheese.
- Payday candy bar, peanut or almond M&M's, or Snickers candy bar in a pinch if none of the above are available; their ratios are not so bad compared to other candy bars

Gas stations and airport newsstands are a little easier to navigate, since you can see the nutrients, but usually you are in a hurry and don't have a lot of time to dwell on the details. Let's go over some possible items that are good options:

- Nuts—mixed nuts, walnuts, almonds, and pumpkin seeds are great options! Not all nuts are created equal, so look at the labels and choose wisely.
- Trail mix—since you can see the nutritional content, take the time to check out the ratios of dietary fat, protein, and carbohydrates before deciding on a trail mix. If there is one that you like and you can omit eating some of the raisins and most of the dried fruit, then go for it!
- Beef jerky—definitely a good bet
- Protein bar—check out the ratios of dietary fat, protein, and carbohydrates. Many "protein" bars offer very little protein in comparison to the carbohydrate and fat contents. The source of protein may be soy, which has been thought to affect thyroid function, so be very careful!

Nice Sit-down Restaurant

Appetizers—share unless you are at a restaurant that provides individual portions

- Oysters on the half shell (easy on the red or white sauce—the clear sauce is a better option)
- Shrimp cocktail (easy on the red sauce—with lemon juice or just plain is also delicious)
- Chicken wings (easy on the sauce or forgo the sauce)
- Sushi (do not eat all of the rice—get sashimi if available)
- Goat cheese on Baguettes

- Carpaccio (raw meat—amazing) usually comes with parmesan cheese and greens, and capers
- Smoked salmon (easy on the white sauce and pita crackers)

Salads—most salads are good, but hold the croutons and dried fruits

- Spinach with goat cheese
- Caesar—go ahead and have the anchovy; try *one* if you haven't before
- Iceberg wedge with blue cheese and bacon

When ordering salad out at a restaurant, do *not* ask for your dressing on the side. Instead, ask for easy dressing; this means they will put less on, and you have a greater chance of having the dressing all over the salad and not just in one area. Creamy dressings are more likely to be put on the top, whereas oily dressings are apt to be mixed throughout the salad.

Soups—are trickier

Soups can fill you up fast; only have a cup (not a bowl) no matter what you pick. Do not feel compelled to eat the entire cup. Some soups have a lot of carbohydrates and/or dietary fat, so pick wisely.

Soup options by themselves

- Lobster bisque (with real chunks of lobster)
- French onion (do not eat all the bread at the bottom!)
- Chicken tortilla soup (sans tortilla!)
- Beef with vegetable
- Clam Chowder

Soup options to combine with an entrée

- Tomato
- Vegetable
- Bean
- Pea

Entrées

Almost anything at a sit-down restaurant is a good option, as long as it is not fried, breaded, or crusted. If you have the choice between pasta and vegetables, choose the vegetables if you are in weight loss mode. If you are in maintenance mode, see if you can have a little of each or split with someone else.

Desserts—It is not necessary or always in your best interest to eat dessert

- Dense chocolate cake
- Flourless espresso cake
- Strawberries—À la mode

Mexican Food Restaurants

In my home town of Phoenix, Mexican food is our guilty pleasure. When I was a child we would go every Friday night. Even when raising my daughters we would go several times a month. This is a tradition I did not want to forgo when I was in weight loss mode. So this is what I did. When the salsa and tortilla chips came out, I would take a specific amount of them from the bowl and put them on my plate so as to make sure I knew exactly how many I was eating. I would also make sure I had my own salsa so I could double-dip and make the most of each tortilla chip that I did eat. I drank plenty of water and decided to forgo the margarita.

When it came time to order I would get one or two enchiladas chicken and/or cheese. Then when dinner came I would eat the shredded lettuce and diced tomatoes (that come with every Mexican food dinner) along with my enchilada(s). I enjoyed the time with my friends and family and I did not overeat.

Restaurant Ideas to Make at Home

I always look for menu ideas to make at home. You can eat at restaurants, but you will find that you eat a lot more often than you are used to. It not convenient to go out every time you are hungry; it also can be costly to go out to eat five to six times a day. Here are some of my favorite restaurant inspired ideas.

Breakfast

- Huevos rancheros with chorizo added
- Eggs with beef or ham steak and half an English muffin with butter
- Eggs benedict—this takes a great mastery of cooking
- Smoked salmon with Neufchâtel cheese, diced hard-boiled eggs, red onions, and capers

Mini-Meals

- Crackers with plain goat cheese and salsa on top
- Salami rolled up with mozzarella cheese

Lunch/Dinner

- Taco night—have all the fixings in bowls on the table so everyone can make their taco's the way they like—stick to hard shells for yourself

» Baked potato bar—have individual custard dishes for each topping (including freshly made bacon)
» Cobb Salad—any kind of lettuce—any or all of the following chopped up:
» Tomato
» Bacon
» Chicken breast
» Hard-boiled egg
» Avocado
» Black Olives
» Green Onions (scallions)
» Feta or Blue Cheese Crumbles

Food is to be enjoyed, especially while you are losing weight. Try as many new things as you feel comfortable with and write down how you feel after eating something new. These menus are for you and no two people will want or like the exact same thing all the time. You really are creating your own weight loss plan and insuring you will enjoy the journey.

Answers to the Quiz from Chapter 4—Before You Start

Here are the answers to the nutrients from *Chapter 4—Before You Start* from the website of the National Agricultural Library "Food Group." *Foods List.*N.p., n.d. Web. 11 July 2013. <http://ndb.nal.usda.gov/ndb/search/list>.

a) Dietary Fat   b) Carbohydrates   c) Protein

1. Vanilla ice cream—1/2 cup—Item #19095

   b) 15.58 g   a) 7.26 g   c) 2.31 g

2. Egg—One large—Item #01123

   c) 6.28 g   a) 4.76 g   b) 0.36 g

3. Steak tenderloin—4 oz.—Item #13442

   c) 31.26 g   a) 12.6 g   b) 0.00 g

4. Fresh strawberries—1 cup whole—Item #09316

   b) 11.06 g   c) 0.96 g   a) 0.43 g

5. Whole milk–3.25% milk fat—1 cup—Item #01211

   b) 11.66 g   a) 7.98 g   c) 7.69 g

6. Potato chips–plain, salted—1 oz.—Item #19411

   b) 14.4 g   a) 10.32 g   c) 1.86 g

7. Beef jerky—1 large piece—Item #19002

   c) 9.41 g   a) 7.26 g   b) 3.12 g

8. Salsa—½ cup—Item #06164

   b) 8.74 g   a) 0.22 g   c) 0.20 g

9. Cheddar cheese—1 oz.—Item #01009

   a) 9.4 g   c) 7.06 g   b) 0.36 g

10. Fresh broccoli—1 cup raw—Item #11090

   b) 6.04 g   c) 2.57 g   a) 0.34 g

Appendix D

Exercise

Exercise should become a part of your everyday life, something that you enjoy and look forward to. It can also be a way to prepare you for activities you want to do in the future, like kayaking, water skiing, or running a marathon. You don't need to do any of *these* activities. But if you have one in mind that you have always thought would be fun, you can use that as motivation by having a purpose for how you choose to workout.

My main purpose for exercise is to relieve stress (aerobic activity). I also would like to have my legs look as good as they possibly can and try to reduce the flabby stuff under my arms. Someday, I would love to water ski or wake board with my grandkids, so I have started focusing on my upper body strength, as well. Over the summer I did a 5K Walk/Run (I *walked* with a friend) but before the walk I focused on using the bike to get my legs ready. If you have a purpose it can make the time go faster and become more meaningful.

One caution about exercise is *always* trying to exercise. You may come to resent exercise if you feel you must always be doing something to exert yourself. Sometimes just *being* is great! Pick the amount of time you will work out each day and then live your life. If there are opportunities to take the stairs or walk a little farther and they seem safe and easy enough to incorporate into your life—go for it—if not, then don't! And do not feel guilty about it.

Warm-up and Cool-down

Your warm-up and cool-down are important and do not need to be lengthy in order to be effective. Lightly stretch (do not bounce) the muscles you will use during your routines. For example, if you will work out your biceps and triceps, gently stretch them before *and* after your workout. The stretch does not need to be long; 10–15 seconds is good. Current wisdom is that your cool-down is more important than your warm-up; however, I feel both are important.

Arms

- Bicep stretch
    - Hold one arm straight in front of you
    - Turn the arm so your palm is facing upward
    - With your other hand ***gently*** take your fingers of your arm that is straight out and ***very slowly*** pull them down—this may be only an eighth of an inch or less.

You should feel a stretch but not a pull. Hold for 10 seconds and then do the other arm.

- › Repeat if necessary

» Tricep stretch

- › Take both arms and have them straight up over your head
- › Take one arm and lower it to the closest shoulder behind your head
- › Take the other arm and have it touch the elbow of the arm that is on your shoulder—the forearm holding the shoulder should automatically fall toward the middle of your back
- › Now take the arm that is at the middle of your back and create resistance (***ever so slightly***) at the elbow away from the other arm holding it. Hold for 10 seconds and then switch arms.
- › Repeat if necessary

Legs

» Walking or marching in place at a slow to moderate pace is a great warm-up and cool-down for the legs

There are other more advanced stretches that can be used, but I only want to provide the simplest methods here.

Machines that incorporate warm-ups and cool-downs

When using equipment like a treadmill, elliptical, stationary bike, or stair stepper, you are warming up when you start at a slow pace and then move to a faster pace. For example: on a treadmill, start no faster than 1.5 miles per hour and then increase two-tenths of a mile until you are at a steady but very moderate pace (for me this is 2.2 miles per hour) keep this pace for a full two minutes as part of your warm up. Then increase your speed gradually until you reach the pace for which you feel comfortable. You can increase the pace at any time in your routine if it seems too easy. Never go so fast that the pace is uncomfortable, makes you feel uneasy, or out of breath.

When you are done with your treadmill workout, reduce the miles per hour by two-tenths of a mile until you are back down to your moderate pace (again mine is 2.2 miles per hour). Keep the pace for about two minutes for your cool-down (longer if needed—you should be breathing normally when you step off the machine). Never skip your warm-ups or your cool-downs.

How to Use the Journal

Aerobic activity can be done every day, but weight resistance on your arms and legs should be done on alternating days. There are journals you can set up manually using the forms at *www.timerdiet.com/journals*. Also, there is a website that links to the *Timer DIET* Apps using the *Member Portal* at *www.timerdiet.com/login* or download the App to your Android or Apple device.

Put a check mark next to the exercises you are going to do (if you do not have time to do them all). You do not want to think about your next set in the middle of your routine and you want all muscle groups included. Calculate how many sets you will do based on how long you are devoting to the entire routine. Normally you will want to complete a set three times using different weights. This is not an absolute rule, especially if you are short on time—doing only one or two sets is better than none!

For example, you have 15 minutes to work on weights—today we are doing arm weights. I would pick 5 exercises (15 minutes divided by 3 sets). Then I would check off two tricep exercises (my weak spot), biceps, shoulders, and back. And I set my timer for 30 second intervals (for each arm—if both arms are used simultaneously then go through 2-30 second intervals), for a total of 15 minutes—you will not stop in between each set. You are not over exerting yourself; there is no need to stop in-between workouts.

Change your routine every few weeks, including increasing weights as needed and different exercises. (You can rotate back in those exercises you are particularly fond of.) You will probably start out using one and three pound weights when you begin weight training. Start with the weight you feel comfortable with and be sure to increase and decrease your weights throughout your routine. You will not be using the same weight for each exercise or each set. Have at least three consecutive weights available before you begin your workout. Do not hesitate to increase your weights, if you are ready! When doing three sets the last set will not be as much weight as you lifted for your first or second sets—do not workout to the point of fatigue. You are not body building! There are plenty of books on that topic you should read, if you are.

Here is an *example* 15 minute routine (without the warm-up and cool-down):

Set Number One (one minute for each or 30 seconds each arm)

- Dumbbell kickbacks (tricep)—4 lb. weights
- Chest press (shoulder and back)—4 lb. weights
- Concentration bicep curls—5 lb. weights
- Overhead tricep extension—5 lb. weights
- Dumbbell rowing (back and biceps)—5 lb. weights

Set Number Two (one minute for each or 30 seconds each arm)

- » Dumbbell kickbacks (tricep)—5 lb. weights
- » Chest press (shoulder and back)—5 lb. weights
- » Concentration bicep curls—8 lb. weights
- » Overhead tricep extension—8 lb. weights
- » Dumbbell rowing (back and biceps)—4 lb. weights

Set Number Three (one minute for each or 30 seconds each arm)

- » Dumbbell kickbacks (tricep)—3 lb. weights
- » Chest press (shoulder and back)—3 lb. weights
- » Concentration bicep curls—3 lb. weights
- » Overhead tricep extension—3 lb. weights—doubled
- » Dumbbell rowing (back and biceps)—3 lb. weights

Start out with the weight you feel comfortable with and then gradually increase every week or two. There is nothing wrong with starting out with every set at one pound—just give it a try, if you have never done so.

Creating your own workout routine without weights

Sometimes you do not feel like using weights; perhaps you want something more aerobic in your routine at home. Create your own sets—pick one arm exercise and one leg exercise; feel free to mix them up. Set your timer from 1-5 minute intervals, so you don't have to stop in between. I have them in the order which I like to do them. Feel free to do them while watching TV or listening to music—it will make the time fly!

Standing exercises—your hands should be making a semi-relaxed fist at all times and your legs should never go higher or farther than you feel comfortable

Exercise Number One

- Arms forward and back
    - Have both arms at your side and bent at elbow each making an L-Shape
    - Simultaneously move them straight and forward in front of you
    - Return to L-Shape at your sides—continue this motion back and forth
- Legs bent and back
    - Stand straight with your legs shoulder-length apart
    - Pick up one leg and bend it back at the knee and put it down
    - Pick up the other leg and bend it back at the knee and put it down
    - Then alternate

Exercise Number Two

- Arms bent to side up
    - Have both arms at your side and bent at elbow each making an L-Shape
    - Simultaneously have the L-Shape of your arms go up so they are even with your shoulders
    - Return to L-Shape side and repeat
- Leg side step
    - Stand with your feet close to each other—only a couple of inches apart
    - Take one leg and move it so that it is now shoulder length apart
    - Bring the other leg close to the leg you just moved so they are now only a couple of inches apart again
    - Repeat in the opposite direction and then back and forth

Exercise Number Three

- Arms bent and twist at waist
  - Have both arms at your side and bent at elbow each making an L-Shape
  - Simultaneously have the L-Shape of your arms go up so they are even with your shoulders
  - Keep arms steady and twist back and forth at waist
- Legs high march
  - Stand with legs comfortably apart as in a marching stance
  - Lift one leg at a time by bending at the knee as high as possible
  - March in place

Exercise Number Four

- Arms swinging
  - Have both arms at your side and bent at elbow each making an L-Shape
  - Alternate bringing the L-Shape of your arms straight up like you are undercutting (a boxing term)
- Legs fast march
  - Stand with legs comfortably apart as in a marching stance
  - Lift one leg at a time by bending at the knee—not high
  - March in place

Standing exercises as a set

- Arms bent one at a time, lower to opposite knee raised up
  - Have both arms at your side and bent at elbow each making an L-Shape

    - Keep arms steady and lower them retaining their L-Shape while raising one of your legs between your arms
    - Stand with legs comfortably apart as in a marching stance
    - Lift one leg at a time by bending at the knee as high as possible
    - Lift each leg alternating to be between your L-Shaped arms
- Arms down touching elbow to knee alternating
    - Have both arms at your side and bent at elbow each making an L-Shape
    - Simultaneously bring the L-Shape of your arms straight up like you are undercutting (a boxing term) and hold
    - Lift your right leg to touch your left elbow that is in a hold position (bend it down a *tiny bit* if needed—if you cannot comfortably touch your knee to your elbow do not do this exercise—yet)
    - Alternate your left leg to touch your right elbow

Laying down exercises—these can be done instead of weight training on your legs

- Lie on the floor on your side and raise outer leg (high but not hurting)
- Lie on the floor on your side and raise inner leg (not as high)
- Lie on your back and pretend to bicycle in the air (if you feel the slightest strain in your back then either put your hands underneath your buttocks to provide some lift or a small pillow)
- Lie down on your back and bring your knees up so that your

legs are creating an upside down L-Shape. Keep your toes touching and separate your knees away from each other and then bring them back together. You will probably feel more comfortable with your hands behind your head. You should feel this in your inner thighs—do not add any extra weights to your legs (if you feel the slightest strain in your back put a small pillow under your buttocks)

» Sit in a sturdy chair and raise legs at knees—alternating each leg

Push-ups—an amazing way to get your entire upper body in shape

» Easy—push yourself against a sturdy wall
» Beginning—bend at your knees and push from the floor
» Intermediate—on your toes and push from the floor
» Advanced—variations of the intermediate including using one handed push-ups

Video workouts—I have to admit my favorite workouts were on VHS— and are nowhere to be found in the digital world. The new ones are good, but nothing like what we used to have available to us.

Look at each video and see how much time in total each routine will take you. Some are very long and if you do not have the time to do the entire workout including the warm-up and the cool-down, you risk injury. So be sure the video selected fits the time you have allocated. Some great *types* of video's are:

» Boot camp
» Kickboxing
» Step aerobics
» Dance

Enjoy What You Do

It may be unrealistic to enjoy working out at first, since you may not be used to it. You may associate working out with doing a chore or consider exercise a necessary evil in the role of weight loss. But if you learn to appreciate all of the positive effects of exercise, you will realize that exercise is not so much about weight loss as it is about overall health and well-being. Embrace it as something that you want to partake in for the rest of your life.

Try to find things to do that you enjoy—or at least you think you will enjoy—like hiking, swimming, racquetball, riding a bike, or dancing. Have a "Let's give it a try" attitude. If you like it, then incorporate it into your routine; if you decide you don't, then don't!

In Conclusion

Now you know you were able to lose the weight and keep it off without lotions, potions, or pills and without much fanfare. Maybe you are saying, "That wasn't so bad after all!" That's the point—it wasn't so bad after all! You make your goals (long-term and short-term), obtain the skills and knowledge to be successful, come up with a plan, and adjust as needed along the way. You keep your momentum—continuing to move forward, and figure out ahead of time what you will do when you succeed in order to keep the success you have worked so hard for.

There is so much more to life than worrying about your weight, and now that you don't have to, the possibilities are endless. The availability of your time and energy to focus on something new, right now, could not be better. Take the time now to create your *new* journey. Write down all the things that you wanted to do but thought you were too young, too old, not the right time, so out there people would judge you and look at them again. Ask yourself, "What if? What if I did it anyway, despite all the obstacles? How would my life be different?" I pray you get your answer; I have a feeling that you will.

Sherri Sue Fisher